Vital Notes for Nurses: Psychology

Vital Notes for Nurses

Vital Notes for Nurses are indispensable guides for student nurses taking the pre-registration programme in all branches of nursing.

These concise, accessible books assume no prior knowledge. Each book in the series clearly presents the essential facts in context in a user-friendly format and provides students and qualified nurses with a thorough understanding of the core topics which inform professional practice.

Published

Vital Notes for Nurses: Accountability
Helen Caulfield
ISBN: 978-1-4051-2279-5

Vital Notes for Nurses: Health Assessment
Edited by Anna Crouch and Clency Meurier
ISBN: 978-1-4051-1458-5

Vital Notes for Nurses: Professional Development, Reflection and Decision-making
Melanie Jasper
ISBN: 978-1-4051-3261-9

Vital Notes for Nurses: Principles of Care
Hilary Lloyd, Helen Hancock and Steve Campbell
ISBN: 978-1-4051-4598-5

Vital Notes for Nurses: Nursing Theory
Hugh McKenna and Oliver Slevin
ISBN: 978-1-4051-3702-7

Vital Notes for Nurses: Research for Evidence-Based Practice
Robert Newell and Philip Burnard
ISBN: 978-1-4051-2562-9

Vital Notes for Nurses: Promoting Health
Jane Wills
ISBN: 978-1-4051-3999-1

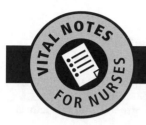

VITAL NOTES FOR NURSES

Psychology

Sue Barker

SEN(M), RMN, BSc, MSc, PG Dip Prof Dev (PCE)
Senior Lecturer
Bournemouth University

Blackwell
Publishing

Blackwell Publishing editorial offices:
Blackwell Publishing Ltd, 9600 Garsington Road, Oxford OX4 2DQ, UK
Tel: +44 (0)1865 776868
Blackwell Publishing Inc., 350 Main Street, Malden, MA 02148-5020, USA
Tel: +1 781 388 8250
Blackwell Publishing Asia Pty Ltd, 550 Swanston Street, Carlton, Victoria
3053, Australia
Tel: +61 (0)3 8359 1011

First published 2007 by Blackwell Publishing Ltd

ISBN: 978-1-4051-55205

Library of Congress Cataloging-in-Publication Data

Barker, Sue, SEN(M)
Psychology / Sue Barker.
p. ; cm. – (Vital notes for nurses)
Includes bibliographical references and index.
ISBN-13: 978-1-4051-5520-5 (pbk. : alk. paper)
ISBN-10: 1-4051-5520-5 (pbk. : alk. paper)
1. Nursing.   2. Nursing–Psychological aspects.   3. Psychology.
I. Title.   II. Series.
[DNLM: 1. Nursing Care.   2. Psychology.   WY 87 B255p 2007]
RT86.B36 2007
610.7301'9–dc22

2006102877

A catalogue record for this title is available from the British Library

Set in 10/12pt Palatino
by SNP Best-set Typesetter Ltd., Hong Kong
Printed and bound in Singapore
by Markono Print Media Pte Ltd

The publisher's policy is to use permanent paper from mills that operate a
sustainable forestry policy, and which has been manufactured from pulp
processed using acid-free and elementary chlorine-free practices. Further-
more, the publisher ensures that the text paper and cover board used have
met acceptable environmental accreditation standards.

For further information on Blackwell Publishing, visit our website:
www.blackwellnursing.com

Contents

Preface

This introductory text for nurses provides a foundational understanding of psychology applied to nursing care. It is aimed at pre-registration nursing students but may be useful for those seeking to undertake a nursing course. There are seven chapters, the first of which offers a preliminary insight into the different perspectives in psychology; these then underpin the topics in the other chapters.

I believe this introduction is useful to nurses at the beginning of their career, and it relates closely to some of the psychology units that have been developed by the psychology team in nursing at Bournemouth University.

I have been lecturing psychology to nurses since February 1998, both before and after they have become registered with the Nursing and Midwifery Council. I have also worked as a mental health nurse since January 1983. Over the years I have been supported by my colleagues, both clinical and academic, in my psychological understanding of the people I care for. More recently I have found that the student nurses who I endeavour to teach have become a major source of my learning.

Without the support and encouragement of colleagues, academic, clinical and administrative, supervisors and student nurses, I would not have been able to develop this book and I am extremely grateful to them.

The majority of my gratitude needs to go to my forever tolerant family: my husband Julian, the most tolerant man I have ever met and without him I would not be me – perhaps Erikson was right about women's stages 5 and 6 actually being achieved the other way round; and my children Miriam and Jethro who, whilst tolerating my studies, have continued to stretch my psychological understanding of development and relationships, but without them my life would lack much of its colour.

To develop an understanding of psychological theory I have used numerous examples. I have endeavoured to ensure that any of the examples I have used do not relate to any specific known individuals, therefore any similarities found between names and issues are accidental.

Sue Barker

Fly High, Breathe Deep and Seek Peace

How does Psychology Support Nursing Practice?

Learning Objectives

This chapter introduces the five perspectives of psychology and offers their differing understanding of people and the way they think, feel and behave. It offers an exploration of how the perspectives may gain evidence for their theory and how psychological theory is put to use through different professions. These perspectives provide a basis for the further chapters, which explore different topics related to both nursing and psychology.

- Identify the similarities between nursing and psychology.
- Describe the five perspectives in psychology.
- Identify a variety of research methods.
- Recognise the different roles of psychologists related to health.

Introduction

This chapter briefly explores a range of psychological perspectives considering how each of them may explain elements of a nurse's behaviour. It will explore definitions of psychology and nursing with a view to demonstrating the similarities and differences between the fields but also how the discipline of psychology can enhance nursing practice. The research methods component concisely describes the major research approaches in psychology and offers an example of how each perspective may use the method to explore an area of health that interests them. A brief explanation is given of each of the main psychological professions with which a nurse may come into contact.

As with any scientific approach one question leads to another; if we are to explore how psychology supports nursing practice the first step is to gain an understanding of what nursing practice is and what psychology is.

Activity

Spend a few minutes writing a list of things that you believe a nurse does and then spend a few minutes writing down what you believe psychology is.

Definitions

Nursing

In 1966 Virginia Henderson (cited Siviter 2004) stated:

> *'Nursing is primarily assisting the individual in their performance of those activities contributing to health, or its recovery that they would perform unaided if they had the necessary strength, will or knowledge.'*

The Royal College of Nursing (2003, cited Siviter 2004) defined nursing as:

> *'the use of clinical judgement in the provision of care to enable people to improve, maintain, or recover health, to cope with health problems and to achieve the best possible quality of life whatever their disease or disability until death.'*

Psychology

> *'Psychology is the scientific study of behaviour and mental processes. Behaviour includes all of our outward or overt actions and reactions, such as talking, facial expressions and movements. Mental processes refer to all the internal, covert activity of our minds, such as thinking, feeling and remembering.' (Ciccarelli & Meyer 2006)*

Psychology seeks to understand why people behave, think and feel the way they do, individually and in groups, in all areas of life including health. Psychologists not only seek to predict behaviour but also to change behaviours to enhance well-being and quality of life. This can be seen to link very closely with what nurses do.

Nurses and psychologists seek to understand the health needs of the people they work with but also to change their behaviours, thoughts and feelings to enhance the well-being of the person, not only at this moment but also for the future. At times nurses need to provide very basic care for the people they work with but they are always looking to develop the person's ability to be more independent in any area of their life.

Nurses and psychologists both have strict codes of practice, which guide their work and ensure an ethical approach to their professional practice. Nurses are governed by their professional body, called the Nursing and Midwifery Council (NMC), which has developed a code of conduct for their professional behaviour. Likewise psychologists in Britain are governed by the British Psychological Society, which lays down strict ethical codes for practice and research.

Nurses can use psychological research and theories to enhance their nursing practice, and most nursing practice has a foundation in psychology, sociology or biology. Nursing now has developed its own unique body of knowledge but other sciences can still enhance nurses' understanding and practice.

Psychology perspectives

Psychology has a number of different ways of trying to understand the person and these are called perspectives. These perspectives have changed over the years but the most commonly used now are:

- Biological
- Psychodynamic
- Behavioural
- Cognitive
- Humanistic

Each of these perspectives has a different explanation or theory for a person's behaviour that influences not only psychologists' understanding but also how they conduct research to further this understanding.

Biological psychology

Biopsychologists are often accused of reductionism, which means they reduce the person down to their biological components so explanations of human or animal behaviour are said to be due to anatomy or physiological changes such as chemical reactions in the nervous and endocrine systems. They suggest that biological function and structure determine behaviour; for example people cannot fly because they do not possess wings. A biological understanding of how people behave is crucial for nurses. Without a recognition that a person's biological functioning will affect their behaviour, nurses would have reduced the opportunity for them to offer appropriate interventions.

Case study   Mrs Lillian Child

As a student nurse you are asked to monitor the well-being of an elderly lady, Mrs Lillian Child, who has just been admitted to an assessment ward. Mrs Child appears confused and is agitated and says she wants to go home. Her husband is very worried because her concentration, attention and memory have deteriorated dramatically over the past week. Mrs Child also moans at times as if she is in pain. While monitoring Mrs Child you find her pulse rate is a little raised as is her temperature, breathing and blood pressure. Mrs Child is unable to explain what she thinks is wrong.

The nurse in charge of the unit asks what you think might be wrong with Mrs Child and your mind runs wildly through cancer, anxiety, infection and a number of other options. After a physical examination it is found Mrs Child is constipated, and she is offered an enema to allow some rapid relief. Mrs Child's agitation and mental functioning quickly return to normal for her. She is also prescribed a laxative for a couple of weeks and given information on diet, exercise and her other medications.

Biopsychologists recognise that biological functioning can significantly influence behaviours, which allows for a biological understanding of Mrs Child's confusion and agitation.

Biopsychologists identify biological causes for behaviour and individual differences such as:

- Genes
- Anatomical differences
- Development through the lifespan
- Biological systems such as:
  - the nervous system
  - the endocrine system

Therefore behavioural change could be due to changes in the nervous system, endocrine system, or anatomical or genetic structure. There are numerous factors that could influence this functioning, such as:

- Development and maturation
- Infection
- Mutation
- Nutrition
- Disease
- Trauma
- Environmental factors

Biopsychologists suggest that people develop through a sequence of maturation and growth of the body, including the endocrine and nervous system. Therefore behaviour could be determined in the absence of disorder or disease by the maturational stage of development, genetic makeup, hormonal state and neural readiness.

Genes

Each cell of the human body contains a nucleus. This nucleus usually has 23 pairs of chromosomes. These chromosomes contain the genetic code for the person; it is called DNA (deoxyribonucleic acid). This genetic code provides the genotype for the person, the colour of the hair, their potential height, etc. What is seen of the person is said to be their phenotype; that is, the genotype that has been influenced by the environment.

Box 1.1   Explanation of genotype and phenotype

The genotype for a person may dictate they should be two metres tall (genotype) but due to neglect and malnutrition (biological intervention) the person is not able to fulfil this potential and only achieves a height of one and a half metres (phenotype).

Nervous system

There are two parts to the nervous system: the central nervous system and peripheral nervous system. The central nervous system is made up of the brain and spinal cord, whereas the peripheral nervous system is made up of billions of nerve cells, bundles of which are called nerves.

The peripheral nervous system has three parts:

- Cranial nerves
- Spinal nerves
- Autonomic nervous system

All three communicate information from the senses to the central nervous system and take commands from the central nervous system. The cranial nerves link with the brain, the spinal nerves to the spinal cord and the autonomic nervous system primarily controls the internal organs.

The autonomic nervous system has three components:

- Sympathetic nervous system
- Parasympathetic nervous system
- Enteric nervous system

The sympathetic system prepares the body for action, whereas the parasympathetic system prepares the body for rest. The enteric system regulates the digestive system and is influenced by both the parasympathetic and sympathetic nervous systems.

Endocrine system

The endocrine system is made up of glands that secrete hormones into the body. The major endocrine glands are shown in Table 1.1.

Biopsychologists study how each of these areas influence the behaviour of the person, in their search to understand that behaviour. There

Table 1.1 Endocrine glands and their principal effects. Adapted from Rosenzweig et al. 2005.

Gland	Principal effect
Pineal gland	Regulates seasonal changes and puberty
Hypothalamus	Regulates hormones released from pituitary gland
Pituitary gland	Produces a number of hormones which stimulate growth and development
Thyroid	Involved in metabolism and blood homeostasis
Adrenal glands	Regulates metabolism and body hair. Helps maintain blood sugar level
Pancreas	Involved in the metabolism of sugars
Gonads	Stimulate the development and maintenance of sexual characteristics and behaviour
Stomach	Involved in digestive processes
Heart	Promotes salt loss in urine

is the recognition that the nervous system communicates with the endocrine system and vice versa (see Chapter 7). The chemicals produced by these systems influence each other to achieve this. Neurotransmitters influence the production of hormones as nerves infiltrate the glands and hormones circulate the body changing the chemical environment of the nerves.

Case study   Biological response to stress

A patient observes a nurse coming towards them with a sphygmomanometer to check their blood pressure but do not know what this entails. The patient's eyes perceive this stressor; the information is relayed via the optic nerve (nervous system) to the visual cortex (brain – nervous system) through the thalamus (part of the brain), which in turn passes the information to the hypothalamus (part of the nervous and endocrine system). The hypothalamus triggers the pituitary gland (endocrine system), which releases a hormone (adrenocorticotropic hormone); this activates the adrenal glands (endocrine system), which produce adrenaline. The production of adrenaline has a dramatic effect on the peripheral nervous system and is experienced by the person as stress or panic. The person will either stop the nurse from taking the blood pressure and/or the blood pressure will be raised.

Summary

Biopsychologists seek to understand behaviour from a biological basis, offering biological theories for human behaviour. They identify that people develop through a sequence of maturational changes as the nervous and endocrine systems develop. Nurses too seek to understand behaviour from a biological basis, regardless of the branch of nursing. This is widely viewed as the medical model but it is more useful for nurses to recognise this as one component of the whole person and label it biological.

Psychodynamic psychology

Introduction

This perspective was developed by Freud but a number of theorists have continued to develop his theory, such as Eriksson (see Chapter 4),

Jung and Klein. Sigmund Freud lived from 1896 to 1939 and much of his work has become a significant part of both psychological thinking and western society's thinking. A key component of his theory was around the inner or unconscious conflicts that motivate a person's behaviour. He does, though, suggest that some of these desires or thoughts can become conscious through therapeutic techniques such as 'free association', 'dream interpretation' and 'transference'. Whilst many nurses struggle with viewing people they work with from a psychodynamic perspective, it is already part of their everyday thoughts and understanding of the world.

Box 1.2   Examples of Freudian slips

A man lives with a nagging wife. She is admitted to hospital and quickly recovers from her illness. On seeing her he intends to say, 'I'm glad to see you are better' but what he actually says is, 'I'm sad to see you are better.'

The nurse sees the next patient and instead of saying, 'I can see you now Mr Stanley' says, 'I can see you now Mr Stud.'

These are examples of what are commonly known as Freudian slips (parapraxes). Freud said that all behaviour is meaningful and when people say things that are different from what they intended, their unconscious thoughts are breaking through to consciousness. Freudian slips are part of everyday language in western societies.

Freud developed a structure of the mind, which includes three components:

- Id
- Ego
- Superego

Id
This is the part of personality or mind that a person is born with. It is the largest part of the unconscious structure of the mind. The id holds the sexual and aggressive instincts of the person and demands instant gratification. It is sometimes referred to as the psychic energy.

Ego
This part of the personality or mind is the largest part of the conscious mind but at least half of it is preconscious. The ego develops in

childhood and fulfils a function of balancing the desires of the id with the social constraints of the world which are internalised by the superego.

Superego
The superego is often referred to as the conscience of the person, which is developed at about the age of five. The superego uses guilt and pride to facilitate compliance with social norms. The superego is partly conscious but also exists in the preconscious and unconscious.

Developmental process

Freud also offered a developmental process by which this structure of the personality was achieved. He suggested children are born with the id but develop the ego and superego through psychosexual developmental stages. These experiences in early childhood have a strong impact on the later personality (see Chapter 2).

Freud's stages of psychosexual development are:

- Oral   0–18 months
- Anal   18–36 months
- Phallic   3–6 years
- Latent   6 years to puberty
- Genital   puberty onwards

Freud suggested that the child derives pleasure from different bodily areas at different times of their life. These areas of fascination become the label for the psychosexual stages. If the child successfully progresses though each stage they will develop a full self-concept, but if they are over or understimulated in any area they will be fixated in that area. If a child becomes fixated at a particular stage they will have a certain type of personality (see Chapter 2).

It has been suggested that the most important of these psychosexual stages is the phallic stage; this is where the child experiences either the Oedipus or Electra complex and where the superego or conscience starts developing. It is where the child becomes aware of their own gender and a rivalry develops towards the same sex parent to compete for the affection of the opposite sex parent. Boys and girls resolve this in different ways; the boys identify with the father due to fears the father will castrate them. If children do not identify with the same sex parent, they may go on to develop homosexual relationships. Girls recognise that they do not have a penis and believe themselves to be castrated already, and develop penis envy. Girls go on to change this desire for a penis into a desire to have a baby, preferably a boy baby.

Mental defence mechanisms

The mind as described by Freud is a dynamic structure with continuous conflict between the desires of the id and the social constraints of the superego. The ego attempts to resolve some of these conflicts by the use of mental defence mechanisms. Mental defence mechanisms do not resolve the anxieties or problems but allow the person to perceive them differently.

There is no agreed number of mental defence mechanisms, with some suggesting there are just nine and other proposing 35. However, there is agreement on their characteristics. They are (Stewart 2005):

- Unconscious
- Distinct
- Dynamic
- Can be adaptive or pathological
- Manage instincts, drives and feelings

Summary

Freud offers a psychodynamic theory of the mind, personality and its development. It is a psychosexual theory, which has a number of stages of development. Freud identified the impact that these stages have on the personality and offered mechanisms that the person would use to manage the continuous internal conflict of the different components within the mind. This perspective offers the nurse a completely different way from previous biopsychologists to understand the people with whom they work and themselves. It demonstrates how a person's childhood may have influenced their personality and that this personality rather than being totally fixed is always in a state of movement and tension. It also offers an approach for understanding reactions to health problems that they may experience.

Behavioural psychology

Introduction

The behaviourists are concerned with learning. They propose that all of a person's behaviour, including their personality, is learnt. There are a number of processes by which this happens and they have

Table 1.2 Most commonly identified mental defence mechanisms. Adapted from Gross (2001), p. 624, Table 42.5.

Name of defence mechanism	Description	Example
Repression	Forcing a threatening memory/feeling/wish out of consciousness and making it unconscious	You feel sexually attracted to one of the people you are caring for but force this desire out of your consciousness
Displacement	Transferring feelings from their true target onto a harmless substitute target	One of the other members of the multi-disciplinary team keeps interrupting when you are trying to inform a patient about a health issue, but instead of dealing with them you go home and shout at your partner
Denial	Failing/refusing to acknowledge/perceive some aspect of reality	This can be observed when a patient refuses to accept that they have a serious illness
Rationalisation	Finding an acceptable excuse for some unacceptable behaviour	A client you have been supporting at great emotional expense makes a complaint about the amount of support they are receiving. You feel angry but rationalise their behaviour as being due to their ill health
Reaction–formation	Consciously feeling/thinking the opposite of your true (unconscious) feelings/thoughts	You strongly dislike one of your nursing colleagues so become extremely considerate/polite to them – even going out of your way to be nice to them
Sublimation	A form of displacement in which a substitute activity is found as a way of expressing some unacceptable impulse	You have been trying for the whole shift to make a telephone referral but each time the telephone has been engaged; at the end of the shift you feel very frustrated and so take yourself to the gym
Identification	Incorporating/introjecting another person into one's own personality – making them part of oneself	You are working in the accident and emergency department and a woman comes in who has been raped. When you suggest she speaks to the police she refuses as she believes the man was frustrated and she had encouraged him by wearing revealing clothes
Projection	Displacing your own unacceptable feelings/characteristics onto someone else	You find you are not able to relate to one of your patients and instead of saying you do not get on with them you say that they do not get on with you
Regression	Reverting to the behaviour characteristic of an earlier stage of development	When asked to clean the clinic room for the second time that day you lose your temper
Isolation	Separating contradictory thoughts/feelings into 'logic tight' compartments	A patient has taken their own life but you talk about it without any display of emotion

become the building blocks of learning from the foundational level of habituation to the more complex learning of social learning theory. Habituation can be seen as the lowest form of learning, in that it is a process where the organism becomes 'used to' the presence of a stimulus.

Box 1.3   Example of habituation

A patient review is occurring in a room near a busy railway line where trains frequently go by. Initially you are distracted by the noise but after a little while you habituate to it and do not notice the trains and can concentrate on the review.

Classical conditioning

Learning can also involve association (classical conditioning). This occurs when a stimulus produces a response. This stimulus then gets presented with another stimulus that does not produce that response. After being presented together a number of times, both stimuli can produce the same response. This type of learning is usually considered reflexive learning, where the organism's reflexive responses are being trained.

Box 1.4   Example of classical conditioning

A person who needs pain-killing tablets is given a sugar tablet at the same time. After a number of times with the two types of tablet being presented together, a reflexive association is formed so that the sugar tablet provokes the same response as the pain killer – pain relief.

This type of learning was developed by Ivan Pavlov (1849–1936) when he was studying dogs' digestion. He recognised that dogs could be trained to salivate by pairing or associating another *stimulus* with food. Salivation is a reflex response to food. This reflexive *response* to food was *conditioned* to occur when a bell rang. This theory was then applied to people as well. It was found that pairing one stimulus with another stimulus could also provoke a reflexive response in people. This is also called a stimulus–response theory of learning.

Operant conditioning

Learning also occurs in a more obvious manner where a person will learn that to do one thing rather than another produces a reward (operant conditioning). This can be seen in many animals as well as people.

Box 1.5   Example of operant conditioning

A child is frightened of seeing the nurse because each time they see the nurse an injection is given. The nurse recognises this, and allows the child to play with a stethoscope while administering the injection and gives the child a sticker saying how brave they have been, to wear home. The child is rewarded for their behaviour (allowing the nurse to give them the injection) and they behave less fearfully in the future, in anticipation of a reward.

This type of learning was initially developed by Thorndike (1874–1949) but Skinner (1904–1990) went on to extend this work. He suggested that in the real world animals did not just respond to one stimulus, and he looked at how they operated within their environments (see Chapter 3).

Social learning theory

Another form of learning that builds on the previous levels of learning is social learning theory, which acknowledges a cognitive element to learning. It suggests that learning can occur not only by habituation, association and reward but also by observing others' behaviour and imitating it.

Box 1.6   Example of social learning theory

A relative needs to be informed that their loved one has died. The student nurse observes the experienced nurse giving the relative this information, offering time and support. The student notices how the caring behaviour of the experienced nurse helps the relative, and in the future the student attempts to imitate that behaviour.

Albert Bandura and colleagues developed this theory of social learning through a number of experiments; these demonstrated that observational or vicarious learning could occur without the individual being rewarded. For this type of learning to occur there needs to be an appropriate environment, with another person from whom to learn. This person is usually referred to as the role model. There are five cognitive components that influence the likelihood of learning from a situation:

- Attention
- Memory
- Rehearsal and organisation of memory
- Imitation
- Motivation

Effective role models
There are features that effective role models possess:

- They are rewarded.
- They are similar enough to imitate.
- They are well thought of or respected socially.

Case study   Role modelling with adolescents

Jenny is a children's nurse and is working with a group of adolescents who have recently been diagnosed with diabetes. The young people are anxious about a number of the activities that they need to undertake to manage their diabetes. Jenny is pretty and friendly and dresses in a casual manner; she has a good sense of humour and the young people warm to her. They listen attentively (*attention*), despite attempting to appear not to, because they want to please her (*motivation*) as she explains about the need to monitor their food intake and blood sugar level. They do not like the idea of testing their own blood so Jenny allows them to practise (*rehearsal*) on her and shows them how to read the monitor once a small drop of blood has been gathered. The young people eventually demonstrate their ability to test their own blood (*imitation*) and give themselves their insulin. They are rewarded by Jenny's praise and they reward her by their achievements.

Jenny is a good *role model* because she is similar enough to imitate, they liked her and she was seen to be rewarded by having the job she did and appearing to get on well with everyone.

Summary

There are four key types of learning identified by the behaviourists, although social learning theory does start to incorporate cognitive elements. Each of these theories is highly relevant to healthcare, particularly nursing, not only for the development of the nurses but also to develop the well-being of the people with whom they work. All the theories are built on the principle that all behaviour is learnt. The four types of learning are:

Habituation	the acknowledgement that people can 'get used to' or accept elements in their environment
Classical conditioning	the training of reflexes such as pain by association
Operant conditioning	if good things happen following a behaviour, the person will repeat the behaviour
Social learning theory	nurses can learn from observing and imitating other nurses.

Cognitive psychology

Introduction

The cognitive perspective can be seen as an extension of the behaviourist perspective in that there is an acceptance that behaviour is learnt and that in any situation there is a stimulus and a response. The cognitive psychologists seek to understand what happens between stimulus and response because they recognise that there is not always a predictable automatic response to any given stimulus. There are a number of theorists in the cognitive perspective with a number of developed theories, for example the cognitive developmental theory of Piaget (see Chapter 4).

As the function of the mind and its precise link with the brain are not as clearly defined as with other organs within the body, it is difficult for psychologists to determine how and where information and processing are stored and occur. However, with the growth of technology and research in the area of bio- and neuropsychology, understanding is developing. Therefore cognitive psychologists tend to use metaphors, such as that the brain is an information processing unit like a computer. A computer goes through a logical system every time a problem is initiated. Some cognitive psychologists believe that people do the same thing and liken the brain to the hard drive and the mind to the software.

Activity

Think of the last time you felt unwell and were unsure why you were ill. You probably went through a process of checking what symptoms you have had and what probability there was of you contracting certain illnesses.

You have had aching muscles, your breathing has become difficult, and you have no energy and are tearful. You are aware that there could be a number of reasons for these symptoms, such as if you have been out to night-clubs dancing for a few nights in a row in smoky atmospheres. It might be that you have had a friend with similar symptoms that the GP said was due to glandular fever. Or it might be that you do not understand your symptoms given your environment.

A computer would work methodically through the symptoms and possible causes in a logical manner, ruling out certain possibilities and putting others higher up the list. This is one theory put forward by cognitive psychologists, for human thought and decision-making leading to health behaviours. As you develop a better understanding of health and illness through learning, you become better at attributing causes, as with the GP whom you may choose to visit to gain both diagnosis and treatment.

To choose to visit the GP again may involve a problem-solving approach using a methodical information processing approach.

Key influential areas in the development of the cognitive perspective are (Anderson 2000):

- Information theory
- Artificial intelligence
- Linguistics
- Neuroscience

Information processing approach

The information processing approach is the main paradigm used with cognitive psychology, to understand how people think. It is proposed that thinking is conducted in a process, with some psychologists offering a simple process but others more complex. It is where people mentally manipulate what they know about the world. Components of this approach would include:

- Set processing rules (organised ways in which information is gathered, stored, worked on and used).

- A storage facility for information (memory).
- A central processing unit which manipulates the information (a place where the information is worked on or with).

This information processing approach could include a costs–benefits analysis as a means of problem solving.

Box 1.7   Costs–benefits analysis

A patient with cancer is prescribed chemotherapy to halt the progression of the disease. The chemotherapy's side effects cause the person to feel very unwell. Patients have the right to refuse treatment. The person uses a costs–benefits analysis to decide whether to take the chemotherapy. They weigh up all the benefits of taking the treatment – possible prolonged life etc. – and all the costs of taking the medication, which include the side effects. The person then makes a decision. This is an information processing theory and is called costs–benefits analysis.

Schema theory

Schema theory is a cognitive theory of how people might store information – memory. It is suggested that new information is attached or becomes part of existing memory. A schema is a collection of information on a certain topic/area/thing. It has a fixed component but also has a flexible component.

Box 1.8   A schema

A schema for giving an injection would have fixed components:

- Needle
- Syringe
- Person to give injection to, etc.

But it could also have flexible components:

- What medication is being injected
- Which part of the person the injection is being given into
- Environment in which injection is being given, etc.

These schemas can also be interrelated, so that thinking about one schema can lead to a memory of information in another schema. For example, a giving an injection schema may lead to a health and safety schema.

Cognitive development theory

Jean Piaget (1896–1980) created a theory of cognitive development. Unlike the behaviourists, Piaget suggested that children of different ages thought in a qualitatively different way from adults. His theory was built on a schema theory. He suggested schemas were developed through a process of *assimilation* and *accommodation*.

Assimilation	process of incorporating new information into existing schemas
Accommodation	occurs when new information cannot be assimilated, at which point a new schema needs to be developed.

Using this process Piaget identified four stages of cognitive development; stage one also has six sub-stages:

- Sensori-motor stage   0–2 years
  - Exercising reflexes
  - Primary circular reactions
  - Secondary circular reactions
  - The co-ordination of secondary circular reactions
  - Tertiary circular reactions
  - Invention of new means through mental combinations
- Preoperational stage   2–7 years
- Concrete operations   7–12 years
- Formal operations   12 onwards

At each of these stages children think in quite different ways. They move from one stage to another through a maturational process. In the first stage the baby is concerned with developing physical schemas in its attempts to understand the world. This leads to the second stage where the child is developing internal, symbolic schemas such as language. In the third stage the child is working within the concrete world but has a greater understanding of this and can manipulate it. In the fourth stage the child is developing its ability to understanding abstract terms (such as algebra) and use its imagination.

Box 1.9   Example of Piagetian concept of egocentrism

You are caring for a man who has a four-year-old child; the mother and child are observing you and your interactions with the child's father. You ask the father how he is feeling and the mother turns to the child and asks, 'How does daddy feel?' The child replies, 'Daddy is happy because I ate a biscuit.' The mother explains that the child was allowed a biscuit while they were waiting for you to arrive. Piaget would explain that the child could not interpret what her father felt and so could only offer how she felt herself, which is typical of the preoperational stage of development. This Piaget labelled ego-centrism.

There have been a number of criticisms of Piaget's work but it continues to be influential (see Chapter 4).

Summary

The cognitive psychologists offer a number of differing theories on how people think. This includes people's ability to communicate, attend and remember things. The information processing approach is the most common cognitive approach, whereas the schema theory is the most widely accepted theory of how information is stored. Piaget offers an explanation of how a child develops adult thinking. Cognitive psychology has had a big impact on health psychology. This in turn has been influential in the development of health promotion, which is now a crucial part of a nurse's role. Cognitive psychology offers an explanation for how people make decisions about their behaviour, including health behaviour.

Humanistic psychology

Introduction

The humanistic movement started in the 1950s in response to the mechanistic approach taken by the behaviourists and the conflict and distress focused on by the psychodynamic psychologists. Whilst they accepted that learning was important, they also acknowledged the importance of innate potential and unconscious processes. Their focus was much more optimistic, identifying that the person was an individual, whole being with unique potential, and they offered a spiritual element to psychological theory. They suggested that all people are moving towards self-actualisation to achieve their potential. Unfavourable environments sometimes disrupt this.

Activity

Nurses are expected to provide individualised care recognising the holistic needs of the person.

With this in mind what do you think should be the priorities when conducting an assessment of the health needs of a person?

Maslow

Abraham Maslow developed the hierarchy of needs in 1954. He suggested that people are motivated to fulfil their needs: the motivation to fulfil lower level needs are deficiency drives, which maintain our health, and the motivation to fulfil higher level needs are growth or being drives. Both drives are leading the person to self-actualisation, which can be seen as a rapturous moment or peak experience. Maslow suggested that people have to work their way up from the bottom of this hierarchy to the top (see Figure 1.1) and they could not move to the next level until the needs of the previous one had been fulfilled (see Chapter 2).

> **Activity**
>
> Look at your priorities in your holistic assessment of the health needs of a person. Are they the same as Maslow's? If not, why not?

Rogers

Carl Rogers developed a person-centred approach. As with other humanists he believed that each person was unique; they were able to reach their own potential as long as they were given the right environ-

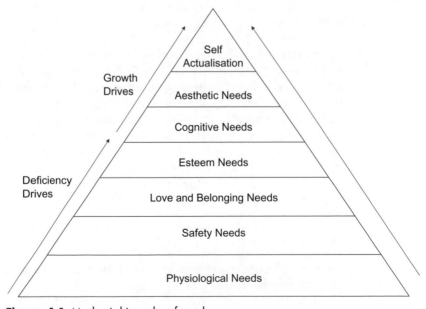

Figure 1.1 Maslow's hierarchy of needs.

ment in which they could grow towards self-actualisation. He developed a theory of self-concept which incorporated the actual self and the ideal self, and he suggested that if these two views of the self were distant from each other, a person would experience psychological distress. To gain a close ideal and actual self, a person needs unconditional positive regard. He went on to develop client-centred therapy to enable people who had not experienced this.

Carl Rogers (1957), who developed client-centred therapy, identified that there were necessary and sufficient conditions for a therapeutic relationship to facilitate change. These are:

- Two people need to be in psychological contact.
- The client is in a state of incongruence.
- The counsellor is congruent.
- The counsellor experiences unconditional positive regard for the client.
- The counsellor has an empathetic understanding of the client and endeavours to communicate this to the client.
- The counsellor is at least successful in communicating unconditional positive regard and empathetic understanding to the client.

Box 1.10 Explanation of client-centred therapy terms

A person you are working with is distressed and not coping with a recent health problem (*incongruent*). As a nurse you need to demonstrate that you are not distressed yourself (that you are *congruent*), that you have high regard for the person regardless of who they are (*unconditional positive regard*) and that you can make them aware that you understand how they are feeling (*empathy*) and care about them.

Summary

The humanistic perspective is a collection of diverse theories, but they have similar underlying principles. These are that:

- The person is motivated to self-actualise – they have the desire to achieve their potential.
- The person is unique – each person is different.
- The person has unique potential – each person has a different set of abilities and they have an individual sense of fulfilment.
- People need positive regard to remain healthy – to be acknowledged as having intrinsic value is important for well-being.

Section summary

This section has explored the main five psychological perspectives. An overview of the most significant areas of exploration from each perspective's theory has been offered: the biopsychologist's search for links between brain and behaviour, the behaviourist's view of the centrality of learning, the cognitive psychologist's exploration of thought, the psychodynamic view of the mind, and the humanist's attempts to understand a person's sense of meaning. Each perspective is different and offers nurses differing perceptual insights into the people that they care for and work with.

Research methods in psychology

Introduction

There are a number of research methods used in psychology. Each perspective tends to use different approaches to research, depending on how they believe understanding can be gained. Research is a scientific way of gaining understanding. The perspective the psychologist adheres to will influence what they are trying to understand, which in turn influences how they try to gain that understanding.

Experiments or quasi-experimental methodology

This method is accepted by the physical sciences to be valid, with the ability to be rigorously tested. The biological psychologists may use this methodology along with the cognitive and behavioural psychologists. It is where all unnecessary variables are eliminated from the experiment, except the things pertaining to the question or hypothesis. This approach is frequently conducted in research laboratories where distracting noises etc. can be stopped. A criticism that may be offered by the humanistic or psychoanalytic perspectives is that it offers little insight into how people behave in the 'real world', i.e. it lacks ecological validity.

Box 1.11   Example of quasi-experimental research

A biological psychologist may be interested in whether nurses who are working night shifts make more drug errors than nurses working during the day owing to their blood sugar level. They would need to set up a question or hypothesis such as 'nurses who work at night make more drug errors than those who work during the day owing to low blood sugar'. This hypothesis would be tested by setting up an experiment (test) where perhaps a number of nurses were recruited and were given drug calculations to do under laboratory conditions. They would all be tested at the beginning to ensure that they all had similar test scores originally, or poor and high scorers could be matched so that those doing the tests at nights had the same average ability as those doing the tests during the day. Each time the nurses took a drug calculation test, their blood sugar level would be monitored as well. The scores of those doing the drug calculations, and their blood sugar levels at night and during the day, would be compared using statistical analysis.

Individual case studies

This method of research can be, and has been, used by all the perspectives but is favoured by the psychoanalytic and humanistic perspectives. A single person's experience is explored in detail, usually by interviewing them or getting them to keep a diary, which could be verbal, written or video. A criticism of this that is put forward by the biological and cognitive psychologists would be the inability to generalise from the findings; if one person responded in this way it does not provide evidence that others will. The perspectives that use this method may suggest that each person is unique and therefore not open to generalisation. It is a methodology that is used frequently in health services when attempting to understand individual problems.

Box 1.12 Case study method

An individual case study could be conducted to explore a unique experience. A humanistic psychologist may use a description of a person's experience of mental illness to gain understanding of this phenomenon.

This approach has also been used by biological psychologists to understand a person's experience of brain damage, and by behaviourists, as in their experiment with 'Little Albert', where a small boy was conditioned into being fearful of anything white and fluffy by presenting a loud noise each time he was shown a white rabbit (Gross 2001, p. 148).

Surveys/questionnaire research methods

This methodology is used extensively to ascertain attitudes and other such social issues. The biological or cognitive psychologists, all of whom may be interested in generalisable behaviour, may use this method. It is a method for gaining a small amount of information from a lot of people. As with the experimental approach, the data obtained are usually converted into numbers and made sense of by using statistical analysis. A humanist would suggest large surveys add little to the understanding of any given phenomenon.

Box 1.13   Questionnaire method

A cognitive psychologist is interested in why people continue to smoke despite being given the information that it is harmful to their health. They formulate a hypothesis just as the experimenters did, such as 'people smoke despite it being harmful to their health because they do not understand the information about the health risks'. They would then devise a questionnaire to find out if this were the situation, given to a large number of people to ensure gaining a generalisable view.

Observational research methods

This method is used by behaviourists to assess the stimulus-response situations; they observe for antecedents, behaviour and consequences. Biological and cognitive psychologists who may be observing for changes in behaviour also use it. Piaget, who developed the cognitive development theory, used this approach to help develop his theory along with experiments. A large part of a nurse's role is to observe patients and so nurses could be considered to be undertaking research when they carry out this task.

Box 1.14   Observational method

A behavioural psychologist may want to understand why residents in a residential care home for people with learning disabilities become aggressive towards the staff. They would observe and record what is happening before, during and after any aggressive outbursts.

Interviews and focus group research methods

The humanistic, psychodynamic and cognitive researchers may use these methods but would probably use different types of approach to the data collection and analysis.

Box 1.15   Interview and focus group method

Interviews – a humanist may use this approach to gain an understanding of the lived experience of being diagnosed with cancer.

Focus groups – could be used by humanists to gather ideas on how to develop a service to enhance older people's attendance at a daycare centre.

Self-report/diary/self-reflection

This is a method used by many psychologists, including the psychoanalysts (Freud, Jung, etc.), cognitive theorists (Piaget) and humanists (Rogers), but this method tends to be regarded as lacking rigour for the biological and behavioural psychologists, although there are particular occasions where biological psychologists would use this approach, such as individual case studies.

Box 1.16   Diary method

A psychodynamic psychologist, as with a nurse, could use this approach to demonstrate their development from novice to expert therapist/nurse. It could show their learning needs and the impact experiences and teaching had had on them.

Qualitative verses quantitative approaches to research

There is another distinction that needs to be made when considering how psychologists might seek to understand human behaviour: whether to use a qualitative or quantitative approach.

Quantitative approach

This involves measuring behaviour in some way; data would be collected so that they could be counted or measured. Most methods identified above could collect data in such a way as to measure them, but individual case studies and self-report diaries and reflection would not usually be used for this approach. This is the traditional scientific approach to research, with a highly structured method.

Qualitative approach

This approach is seeking a more narrative form of data; it does not seek to measure or count behaviour. Self-report diaries, reflections, interviews, focus groups and individual case studies are more usually used for this approach, but an observational study may also use this approach. It is considered richer and seeks to understand the human experience, and is one more suited to the humanistic and psychodynamic perspectives.

Section summary

There are a number of different ways in which a psychologist can gain an understanding of people and their behaviour. These are called research methods. The research method used by a psychologist is partly determined by their psychological perspective. Research methods fall into one of two approaches: qualitative and quantitative. Nursing research is carried out using the same methodologies as physical science and psychology. They too need to identify whether to use a qualitative or quantitative approach. Nurses do not need to choose their methodology on the basis of their fundamental understanding of the person; according to their perspective they tend to choose a methodology that is most appropriate to the area they wish to understand.

Professions in psychology

Introduction

There are a number of professional fields in psychology, most of which expect further training after a first degree in psychology. These professions are regulated by the British Psychological Society (BPS) in Britain, with their own disciplinary committee and code of conduct (the United States of America and the European Union have their own societies). The BPS also charters psychologists.

Nurses too have different fields or branches within which they work and, as with nursing, in each of these fields or branches there are many different roles. Psychologists in their practice areas and in education may come into contact with many types of psychologists and a few of these are defined here.

Clinical psychologists
Clinical psychologists use the research area of abnormal psychology in their work, and also the areas of health and neuropsychology. They work in many clinical areas such as mental health, child guidance, learning disability, stroke units and rehabilitation units.

Educational psychologists
Educational psychologists are interested in areas such as developmental issues, learning theories and individual differences (intelligence, memory, etc.). Educational psychologists work mainly within schools and assist in providing behavioural programmes for children with psychological needs, which could be developmental, intelligence, memory or disruptive behaviour.

Counselling psychologists
Counselling psychologists are interested in any psychological theories which offer insight into interpersonal helping, skills or understanding. Counselling psychologists work with people to help them understand themselves and psychologically develop.

Forensic psychologists
Forensic psychologists are interested in areas such as individual differences and abnormal psychology, and work with people who have a criminal history. Forensic psychologists provide reports for courts, help solve crimes and also provide treatment for mentally disordered offenders.

Health psychologists
Health psychologists are interested in areas of the interrelationship between theoretical perspectives of stress, personality and attitudes, and use any theoretical perspective that gives insight into people's health behaviours. The role of health psychologists is to develop understanding of health issues to facilitate those who provide healthcare and healthy environments.

Neuropsychologists
Neuropsychologists are interested in the anatomy and physiology of the brain and seek to understand the relationship between structure and process. They attempt to explore areas such as consciousness to aid treatment of people with brain disorder or dysfunction.

Sports psychologists
Sports psychologists are focused on motivational issues and the impact of psychological processes on physical abilities. Their role is to facilitate the person to fulfil their physical potential.

Occupational psychologists
Occupational psychologists are interested in not only motivation but also some of the areas researched by social psychologists, such as attitudes, group dynamics and interpersonal relationships. They assist employers in the recruitment and development of their staff.

Section summary

There are a number of recognised psychologists; this number is continuing to grow and nurses may find themselves working alongside a number of these professionals. Sometimes there is confusion over the difference between psychologists, particularly clinical psychologists, and psychiatrists, probably because they both work closely with people with mental health problems.

Psychiatrists are medically trained; they are qualified doctors who have gone on to specialise in mental illnesses, just as an obstetrician specialises in childbirth. Psychiatrists deal with medical diagnosis and physical treatment. Psychologists are not medically trained, although some may be called 'doctor' due to their research studies. Psychologists working with people with mental health problems work with people to establish what they consider their problems are, and use talking and behavioural therapies to help them.

Nurses work alongside both these professions and are involved in both physical treatments and talking therapies.

Chapter summary

This chapter has considered what nursing practice is and how psychology can enhance nursing. It has offered an overview of the perspectives that structure the science of psychology. Each of these offers nurses the opportunity to develop their understanding of themselves and the people with whom they work. Each perspective accesses different research methods to develop their understanding of people. These research methods are also used by nurses. The final part of this chapter considered the different types of psychologists that a nurse may come into contact with, and recognises that some nurses and psychologists fulfil similar functions in caring for people. As can be seen, there are a number of similarities between psychologists and nurses, and psychological research can enhance nurses' understanding and practice.

Web addresses

British Psychological Society: www.bps.org.uk
Nursing and Midwifery Council: www.nmc-uk.org.uk

References

Anderson J.R. (2000) *Cognitive Psychology and its Implications*, 5th edition. New York: Worth Publishers.

Ciccarelli S.K. & Meyer G.E. (2006) *Psychology*, p. 4. Upper Saddle River, NJ: Pearson Prentice Hall.

Gross R. (2001) *Psychology, The Science of Mind and Behaviour*, 4th edition. Hodder & Stoughton, London.

Rogers C.R. (1957) The necessary and sufficient conditions of personality change. *Journal of Consulting Psychology*, **21**(2), 95–103.

Rosenzweig, M.R., Breedlove S.M. & Watson N.V. (2005) *Biological Psychology, An Introduction to Behavioural and Cognitive Neuroscience*, 4th edition, p. 137. Sunderland, MA: Sinauer Associates, Inc.

Siviter B. (2004) *The Student Nurse Handbook, A Survival Guide*, p. 3. London: Bailliere Tindall.

Stewart W. (2005) *An A–Z of Counselling Theory and Practice*, 4th edition. Cheltenham: Nelson Thornes.

Who is a Nurse?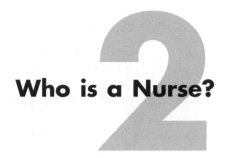

Introduction

This chapter explores the character of the nurse through psychological theory and research. It looks at the implications of working within the nursing field, with identified differences through various theoretical explanations for personality, intelligence, motivation and perception. Initially personality will be explored as an overarching concept, and then the chapter will continue by considering the theoretical approaches to the other individual differences.

Activity

Spend a few minutes writing down what type of person you believe a nurse should be.

- What characteristics should a nurse have?
- What sort of temperament should they have?
- Should they be intelligent?
- What should they look like?
- How should they behave?

At the end of reading the chapter revisit these questions and see if your answers are the same.

Historically nurses have progressed from being considered little more than servants, through the 'lady nurse' such as Florence Nightingale, to the selfless heroine who was kind, patient and cheerful to the healthcare professional of today. The 'underlying socio-cultural context and prevailing system of political power and influence' affects the culture specific image of a nurse that is held today (Fealy 2004, p. 649).

> 'Nurses and midwives can be as diverse in character and temperament as those they'll be helping. Extrovert, shy, ambitious, idealistic; funny, serious. . . . However you think about yourself you probably have the capacity to make a difference in your own life and for others as nurse or midwife' (NHS Careers 2005, p. 3).

This is one standpoint on nurses, but would all characteristics and temperaments be acceptable; those perhaps who are quick to anger or unable to understand treatment regimes, would they too have a place within the nursing profession?

Psychology offers a number of definitions and theories through which to understand individual personalities or characteristics, including those of nurses and the people with whom they work.

One definition of personality is:

> '. . . those relatively stable and enduring aspects of individuals which distinguish them from other people, making them unique, but which at the same time allow people to be compared with each other.' (Gross 1996, p. 744).

If personality is accepted as a starting point for identifying who is, or should be, a nurse, the above definition may be useful. Each of the theoretical perspectives identified in Chapter 1 offers a different understanding of personality.

Personality theories

Psychodynamic

This theoretical perspective is based on the theory of Sigmund Freud who lived from 1856 to 1939. Freud is considered to be one of the great thinkers of the twentieth century. He was a Viennese physician who fled to England to escape the Nazi occupation of Austria (Sternberg 2000, p. 426). He, as with all theorists, will have been influenced by the prevailing socio-political environment of his time, but he may still have something to offer the nurses and psychologists of today.

The term psychodynamic implies that active forces within the personality motivate behaviour, particularly between the three component parts of the personality: id, ego and superego. The id and the superego are largely unconscious and the ego is largely conscious (with some pre-conscious and unconscious components). As with an iceberg, most of the personality lies beneath the surface and therefore cannot be seen.

Case study   Anastasia's interview

Anastasia would like to become a nurse; she has the academic qualifications but she has little care experience, so she has been asked to attend an interview at the university.

At the interview she is asked about any health problems she or her family have had that might have informed her understanding of a nurse's role and what she believes a nurse might do. She is asked why she wants to become a nurse and how motivated she is to study as well as to nursing practice.

While interviewing, the nurse lecturer and senior nurse are also assessing her presentation of herself and her communication skills, both verbal and non-verbal. They are also mindful of attitudes and values she expresses.

Although Anastasia is being assessed for the things she declares and is consciously aware of, she is also being assessed for things that she may be unaware of and unable to verbalise.

Within Freud's theory he describes stages of psychosexual development to attain an adult personality. If a person has problems successfully moving through the three early psychosexual stages, their development may be arrested (fixation), they may return to that stage at times of adult stress (regression) or develop an ongoing personality type linked to that stage. Freud's stages of psychosexual development are as follows.

Oral stage (0–2 years)

At this stage the baby or young child's focus is around the mouth. It is mainly interested in seeking food or stimulation via its mouth, and any new object will be explored orally. If an adult is fixated or regresses to this stage, they are likely to display activities around the mouth: excessive eating, perhaps followed by dieting–excessive eating, drinking, smoking, etc. Two sub-stages of personality types for this stage have been identified.

Oral eroticism
This is where sucking and eating are dominant behaviours and people with an oral erotic personality are likely to be cheerful, dependent and needy.

Oral sadism
For these people biting and chewing predominate and the person is said to be cynical and cruel.

Anal stage (2–4 years)

During the anal stage children are going through a period of toilet training and developing some sense of autonomy, which is usually labelled the 'terrible twos'. This sense of autonomy is linked to the child's recognition that they may have some control over their body through their choosing when to urinate or defecate. The child becomes fascinated with not only their own ability but other people's ability to control their elimination. Two sub-stages of personality types with the anal stage have also been identified.

Anal-retentive
This sub-stage is said to involve the desire to hold on to waste products, and people who regress to this stage or are fixated here are considered excessively neat, clean, meticulous and obsessive.

Anal-expulsive

This sub-stage can be considered the opposite to anal retention and people in this sub-stage tend to be moody, sarcastic, biting and often aggressive. Unlike the other anal stage, these people tend to be untidy in personal habit.

Phallic stage (4 years to middle childhood)

Freud recognises this as a particularly important stage in development; it is when the child struggles with the Oedipal complex, sometimes called the Electra complex in females. Children are said to be recognising their individual sexual identities and through relationships with their parents set the foundations for future sexual relationships. If gender identity is not achieved at this stage, the child may go on to find itself attracted to same sex partners. People who regress to or are fixated in this stage are said to be overly preoccupied with themselves. They are often vain and arrogant and exude an unrealistic level of self-confidence, as well as self-absorption.

Latency (middle childhood)

This is a quiet stage of development according to Freud's psychosexual development. The people fixated or regressing to this developmental stage demonstrate sexual sublimation and repression of sexual desires (see Chapter 1 for mental defence mechanisms).

Genital (adolescence through to adulthood)

This is the final stage of psychosexual development according to Freud, and if the person has not fixated at an earlier stage they will achieve normal adult sexuality and a full self-concept, as defined by Freud (i.e. traditional sex roles and heterosexual orientation).

Case study   Rachel's use of her psychological understanding

Rachel is a student nurse; she is 40 years old and has decided to enter nursing now, as she believes her children are more independent. Rachel has completed some guided study on personality and was particularly interested in Freud's psychosexual theory. Rachel is liked by her peers and always seen as friendly, and people come

Continued

to her when they are struggling; she appears to be a 'mother figure' to her study group. Sometimes this is difficult for Rachel as she too struggles with the academic work and not only has to manage her own time but that of her family as well. Taking responsibility for what appears to her to be everyone has taken a toll on her health.

Rachel's study of the psychodynamic theory of personality has allowed her to gain an understanding of her own behaviours. Rachel can see that when she is finding things difficult she regresses to an oral erotic stage. Her behaviour then becomes overly friendly, she becomes dependent on her children, partner and friends to show her how much they like and need her, and this escalates into needing more acknowledgements, and so she tries to achieve this by being more friendly and helpful, leading to more dependence, etc.

Through this understanding of her personality Rachel is able to halt the spiral and take some time for herself.

Behaviourists

In contrast to the psychodynamic theorists, behaviourists suggest that babies are born solely with the ability to learn. Behaviourists do not recognise a stage theory of development; they suggest that people start learning at birth and continue to learn throughout their lives. They consider that personality can only be assessed by observing individual behaviour; it is a person's behaviour that determines their personality. Personality therefore is learnt in the same way as any other observed behaviour.

- The newborn baby is viewed as a tabula rasa (a blank slate).
- The basis of a given personality is the sum of what is learnt from the environment.
- Behaviour is strengthened by:
  ○ Classical conditioning – reflexive learning by association
  ○ Operant conditioning – learning through reward.
- Behaviour is weakened by punishment (see Chapter 3).

The behaviourists had problems accounting for some unexpected or novel behaviour in people and so this theoretical approach needed to develop new ways of viewing human behaviour. This was achieved through the work of researchers such as Bandura (1965), who established the social learning theory.

Bandura suggested that personality emerges from the interaction between thoughts, the environment and behaviour through:

- Observational learning
- Reinforcement
- Punishment

Bandura's social learning theory allows the behaviourists to account for novel behaviours.

Bandura, whilst accepting the learning processes of classical and operant conditioning, identified through his studies (such as the Bobo doll experiments in 1965) that people learnt through observation and imitation as well. They achieved this through role models. He acknowledged that some role models were more effective than others, for example role models who were socially accepted, were rewarded and were similar in some way to the observer were more likely to be imitated.

Through this process of observation and imitation, called modelling, children develop a self-concept and self-efficacy, which is strengthened in adulthood:

- Self-concept, a collection of thoughts or ideas about oneself, for example, I am a caring person.
- Self-efficacy, the belief in one's own ability to achieve a goal, for example, I am able to dress a wound.

People learn behaviours, including their personality (self-concept and self-efficacy), through modelling. Modelling allows the person to gain attitudes, values and the ability to self-evaluate, which in turn facilitates the person's ability to function in their society. This is seen as the person internalising social standards and expectations, which reduce the need for external reinforcement of behaviour.

Case study   Role modelling facilitating the development of empathy

Paul has just started his first placement on a forensic mental illness unit. Due to learning early in his life, he has developed the moral belief that murder is wrong and that people who commit murder should have their lives taken away from them as well. On his placement Paul meets a woman who has killed her baby. His initial reaction is to avoid her as he has learnt that it is expected of nurses that they behave professionally, which does not include expressing his belief that her life should in turn be taken from her.

Paul's mentor notices his avoidance and encourages him to sit and observe her therapeutic work with the woman. Paul observes the caring, empathetic and non-judgemental approach of his mentor;

Continued

> she is accepting of the woman but at the same time challenging when the woman tries to avoid working on her mental health problem. Through observing the mentor's behaviour, Paul not only learns how to behave but also starts to understand the woman's behaviour. The woman is devastated about what has happened and has little memory of her actions. She knows that she killed her baby but finds it hard reconcile that she believed the thing from which she needed to protect herself was her vulnerable baby.
>
> Paul's attitudes are changing and he is learning to develop empathy and compassion through his mentor (role model).

Trait theories

Two theories of personality have been explored (psychodynamic and social learning theory), and these are considered to be process theories; but there are structural theories of personality known as trait theories. A structural theory of personality identifies personality as fixed and in most cases something a person is born with, and as such, trait theories could be considered biological or genetic theories of personality.

Traits are stable sources of individual differences that characterise what a person is like.

Hans Eysenck (1916–1997) suggested that the personality embraces just three major traits: extroversion, neuroticism and psychoticism. These elements vary within each individual.

Extroversion refers to the extent to which people engage with other people. An extrovert is said to seek proximity to others, whereas at the opposite end of this trait is introversion, which is where people are considered to prefer their own company.

Neuroticism refers to levels of anxiety and worry that a person possesses. A person with high anxiety levels could be considered to have a high level of neuroticism, whereas a person who is more philosophical could be said to possess little of this trait.

Psychoticism refers to how well a person fits in with society, the rules, standards, etc. High levels of psychoticism and the person may be considered deviant; low levels and they may be considered compliant and a rule follower.

Case study   Differing personality traits fulfil differing care needs

Maha and Lee are children's nurses but they have quite different characters. Maha is an extrovert, she has a friendly bubbly approach but she worries about others (high level of neuroticism). It is important to her that she is liked and that those she is working with are happy (low level of psychoticism). She is asked to all the social events of her colleagues and if any of the children need cheering up she is the person who is asked to do this.

Lee though is considered an introvert and is believed to take all situations seriously; he has a calm philosophical approach (low level of neuroticism). He has a few close friends and generally has little in common with the rest of the nursing team (high level of psychoticism).

The nurse manager recognises that Maha and Lee are quite different people but both of them are excellent nurses, with some children and their parents relating better to Maha and others to Lee.

Trait theory of personality could be considered a biological theory in that it suggests people are born with certain traits and essentially maintain these throughout life.

There are other theorists, such as Goffman (1971), who suggest that a person is only the role they are playing at the time. When one is in the role of a nurse one behaves like a nurse, and when one is in university studying to be a nurse one fulfils the role of a student.

Section summary

The psychodynamic, social learning theory and trait theories all offer different understandings of personality, all of which may be useful for nurses in their attempt to assess whether they are the 'right' person to be a nurse or to understand the people with whom they work. Thomas and Chess (1977, cited Sternberg 2000) helpfully suggest that the key determinant of personality is the 'goodness of fit' between an individual's temperament (a nurse's responses) and their environment (situational needs). Therefore to have the personality needed to be a nurse a person has to respond in the expected nurse-like manner to a given situation. This is generally considered to be a caring response. If a person has characteristics that are not considered to be appropriate for nursing, such as being quick to anger, social learning theory and the psychodynamic theories offer the opportunity for the individual to address them to become a nurse.

Intelligence and emotional intelligence

Intelligence was the first area for scientific psychological study of human differences. Initially there were two major approaches, one by Sir Francis Galton (1822–1911) and the other by Alfred Binet (1857–1911).

Francis Galton

Galton believed that intelligence consisted of two general qualities:

- 'Strength' (muscular strength, speed and accuracy in performing tasks)
- 'Psycho-biological ability' (ability to see, hear, taste and touch accurately)

He also believed that if these abilities were measured, they would indicate the intelligence level of the person and predict their future success.

This is a biological view of intelligence, which would indicate that intelligence is due to inherited or genetic factors. These genetic factors could be developed through training. Galton's motivation to study intelligence was influenced by his belief in eugenics. This movement suggested that selective breeding would enhance the human species. Unfortunately for Galton he was unable to provide evidence that his tests predicted future success.

Theodore Binet

Binet's motivation and view of intelligence were quite different. The French Ministry of Education, in the early 1900s, asked him to develop tests to establish the abilities of children to predict and ensure their success. He did this in collaboration with Theodore Simon. The tests they developed could identify high achievers as well as those with some level of learning disability. The tests involved the children making judgements in which they demonstrated practical sense, adaptability and initiative. Unlike Galton, who assumed a biological view of intelligence, Binet's view was more similar to that of the behaviourists.

Later views of intelligence

Sternberg (2000, p. 268) defines intelligence as 'the abilities needed to engage in goal directed adaptive behaviour'.

Gardner (1983, 1993, 1999) over a number of years developed a theory of multiple intelligence. He suggested there are a number of areas in which people can exhibit intelligent behaviour: linguistic, logical–mathematical, spatial, musical, body-kinaesthetic, interpersonal, intra-personal and naturalistic. He went on to suggest that there may also be two further intelligences: spiritual and existential.

Case study   Abe becomes a registered nurse

Abe left school with no formal qualifications and initially worked stacking shelves in a large supermarket. Abe became frustrated with this job; he found it boring and was frequently at odds with his supervisor because he spent too long talking to the customers. He was also approached regularly by his colleagues when they had problems. At one of these moments of frustration his supervisor said why didn't he get himself a different job, as a nurse or something? Abe said he could not become a nurse because he was too stupid and did not have the right qualifications (a Galton or biological theory of intelligence), but he did approach the local Health Trust which sent him information about becoming a healthcare assistant. Abe was interviewed and offered a post.

Abe enjoyed his job, and his manager recognised his potential and ability in communication (interpersonal intelligence), self-awareness (intrapersonal intelligence) and problem solving (logical intelligence). Due to this, Abe was offered the opportunity to undertake a National Vocational Qualification. Abe achieved level 2 and his manager put him forward for secondment to the local university to undertake the diploma in nursing with professional registration. He was accepted onto the course but found the academic work difficult and his personal tutor suggested being tested for a learning disability such as dyslexia. The additional learner-needs department at the university conducted this test for Abe and it was established he had dyslexia.

This was a turning point for Abe as he could now understand the problems he had had during school, and was getting the educational support he needed. Abe went on to gain his nursing registration and an honours degree in nursing. Abe now encourages other people to access education and additional learner support, as he believes anything is possible if you get the right support (a Binet or behavioural view of intelligence).

Emotional intelligence

Mayer and Salovey (1997, p. 10) state that emotional intelligence involves:

> *'. . . the ability to perceive accurately, appraise and express emotion; the ability to access and/or generate feelings when they facilitate thought; the ability to understand emotion and emotional knowledge; and the ability to regulate emotions to promote emotional and intellectual growth.'*

Goleman (1995, p. 160) suggests that for a group to be talented, productive and successful, they need social harmony; this he labels emotional intelligence. Goleman (1995, p. 318) adapted Salovey and Mayer's model of emotional intelligence to address issues of work life and he suggested that there are five basic competencies for emotionally intelligent behaviour in the workplace:

Self-awareness
knowing how we are feeling, what our abilities are and realistic self-confidence

Self-regulation
managing our emotions, delaying gratification if necessary and dealing with personal distress

Motivation
to strive towards goals despite setbacks, moving towards goals based on personal desires

Empathy
Understanding the feelings of a diverse range of other people, using this to gain rapport with them

Social skills
to deal with emotions in relationships, to be able to negotiate with others and develop co-operative relationships, team working skills

Emotional intelligence is considered to be particularly important in nurses. Cadman and Brewer (2001) say that emotional intelligence is a reliable predictor of whether a nurse will be successful both in clinical practice and in academic study. Freshwater and Stickley (2004) go on to highlight that there is an essential need to develop emotional intelligence as a central part of nurse education. They identified that every aspect of nursing is affected by emotional intelligence. They ask, 'What is nursing if it is not the provision of one human being caring for another?' (p. 94), and suggest that this cannot be achieved without emotional intelligence. Despite this strong assertion that emotional intelligence is essential for a nurse, they also recognise the need for a rational technical intelligence, identifying the need for expression of both the art and science of nursing.

Section summary

In this section, theory pertaining to intelligence has been considered. It would appear to be unhelpful to the nursing profession to recognise intelligence as just an innate attribute. It is more useful to recognise a person's ability to learn; this can then be utilised not only to achieve personal success but also to assist others' development through activities like nursing. The ability to learn is important in nursing but there is a lot of literature available that highlights the need for nurses also to be emotionally intelligent.

Motivation

Motivation is another area of individual differences studied by psychologists. It also links to emotional intelligence as expressed by Goleman. Sternberg (2000) states that motivation is an impulse, a desire or a need that leads to action, and Rungapadiachy (1999) suggests it is the energising force of behaviour.

Again, each of the psychological perspectives (see Chapter 1) offers an explanation for motivation.

Biopsychologists

One of the biological theories of motivation is the homeostatic drive theory (Canon 1929, cited Malim & Birch 1998). Homeostasis is derived from the Greek language, homo meaning same and stasis meaning stoppage. Therefore this theory considers the drive to maintain a system or movement and to stop that system or movement.

- The homeostatic drive refers to the internal body processes which work together to maintain a constant optimal bodily environment.
- If the body's temperature becomes higher than is optimal an imbalance will occur and the body will respond to restore its equilibrium.
- Homeostasis regulates, for example, blood pressure, heart rate, digestion, respiration.

Case study   Biological motivation of behaviour

You are caring for Daniel who has cut a major artery and lost a lot of blood, and owing to this he develops hypovolemic thirst (occurs when extra-cellular water is dramatically reduced). Although drinking, like eating, is usually triggered prior to bodily need, in this situation a complicated neural and hormonal reaction occurs. Daniel will be motivated to drink and maybe to eat salty food to achieve bodily homeostasis. Reduction in blood pressure triggers the baroreceptors (found in the walls of blood vessels). This information is passed on to the hypothalamus, which is the main brain structure regulating homeostasis. The hypothalamus releases anti-diuretic hormone (ADH), which reduces the release of water by the kidneys and stimulates drinking behaviour. The low blood pressure also stimulates the kidneys to secrete the hormone renin, which triggers a chain reaction of hormones which eventually constrict the blood vessels. As Daniel continues to bleed, the adrenal

Continued

> glands which sit on top of the kidneys will react to the low levels of salt and release a hormone known as aldosterone. This hormone restricts the release of salts via the kidneys and may increase the motivation to eat salty foods (Green 1994).

People's behaviour, including that of nurses, is motivated by their biological systems and any consideration of who becomes a nurse must take into account the person's biological system, including biological theories of motivation. Whilst they do not offer overarching theories for complex behaviours, they do offer detailed information on specific behaviours, such as the example given, which is important within nurse education. It is important to recognise, as with intelligence, that nurses too may be motivated towards homeostatic behaviours that are not statically normal or average; this does not mean that they would not be able to become nurses.

Psychodynamic

The psychodynamic perspective offers an instinct theory of motivation. Freud initially identified libido as the motivating force for behaviour, which is innate and is found in the id, the pleasure-seeking part of the psyche or mind. This innate drive is in conflict with the learnt morality of the superego (see Chapter 1). Freud later in his life distinguished between two motivational forces: the libido (sexuality) part of the life instinct, or Eros, and the death instinct, which he labelled Thanos. This represented an inborn destructiveness which could reduce inner tension. He also suggested that after being in the womb, the only way to reach Nirvana (peace, lack of conflict) was death (Gross 2001).

Case study   Thanos drive motivating behaviour

You are caring for a young man, Peter, on an orthopaedic ward. It is the third time you have cared for him in the two years you have been working on the unit. He is a bright and cheerful young man and the nursing team enjoy his conversation. Peter on this admission has broken his left leg in a motorbike accident and has been prescribed traction. On his previous admission he had broken his right leg and the admission before that he had broken two ribs, his collarbone and one arm, and both admissions were due to accidents involving his motorbikes (each time he had an accident, his motorbike had to be scrapped). You ask Peter why he does not ride his bike more carefully and prevent himself from getting hurt. Peter explains to you with excitement the great feeling of riding his bike

> at speed round country lanes. The fact that it is dangerous and he may have an accident increases his excitement. This can be understood from a Freudian motivational drive as the desire or motivation to be involved in something that could result in Peter's death.

Whilst the example given here is of a patient, it could just as easily have been a nurse explaining their desire for dangerous excitement. Life and death drives or instincts are said to occur in all people. The management of these is particularly important for those in the caring professions.

Humanistic

The humanists suggest that people have control over their own destiny; they are free agents and able to realise their own potential in their own way. This would suggest that motivation is internal and individual to the person (see Chapter 1).

Abraham Maslow (1908–1970)

Maslow was one of the first of the humanist psychologists and developed the hierarchy of needs, which offers a framework for exploring motivation. Maslow believed that people need to be self-aware and that the ability to come to terms with one's self is necessary for psychological well-being. He suggested that behaviour could be understood in terms of the person seeking to fulfil personal goals to achieve a rewarding and meaningful life. Maslow identified two categories of motive (motivation) or drive – growth and deficiency – and these offer the energising power to achieve personal goals (see Figure 1.1):

- Deficiency motives are those lowest on the hierarchy and move from the biological to psychological; they are physiological, safety, love, belonging and esteem needs.
- Growth motives are those at the top of the hierarchy and promote self-actualisation; they are cognitive and aesthetic needs and self-actualisation (Gross 1996).

Deficiency motives or drives
These are basic needs and if one were missing, the person might become ill; but if the need were fulfilled or restored, it would prevent illness in the person. People are considered to have free will but they would usually prefer to fulfil basic needs rather than other satisfactions. These basic needs are found to be inactive or functionally absent

in the healthy person (Rungapadiachy 1999). These drives are always active in that they continue to exert pressure on the person to fulfil them, as physiological needs such as thirst and hunger can only be satiated for a short period of time. Likewise, as the person is always moving forward, at any moment they may become aware of a safety need. This can become a problem for nurses as they frequently work shift patterns that interfere with the maintenance of these basic needs, which can interfere with their ability to show care. If nurses are aware of these motivations, they can address them and maintain their focus on patient care.

Growth motives

These focus on enriching and expanding one's experience of living. They allow for satisfaction of curiosity, creativeness and ambition. It could be said that growth motives are secondary to deficiency motives (Rungapadiachy 1999). These growth drives can be considered important in nurses as they will motivate nurses to develop and improve their knowledge and skills, which should enhance patient care.

Case study   Using Maslow's hierarchy of needs to understand health behaviours

You are working with a mother, Karen, who is concerned about her daughter Rebecca's health. Rebecca, who is nine years old, eats a balanced nutritious diet, gets ten hours' sleep a night, has a nice home and has regular exercise. Despite this, Rebecca appears pale and lethargic and gets recurrent tonsillitis. Karen does not think that Rebecca is under any particular stress as her siblings are well and happy, Karen has a good relationship with her husband and she believes they have a happy family. You have a conversation with Rebecca about her health and Rebecca says she does not know why she keeps getting ill.

Using your knowledge of Maslow's hierarchy you are able with Rebecca and her mother to discount the lowest levels of need. On further discussion you find that Rebecca, despite having a close family, has few friends at school and feels as if she does not belong to any friendship group (love and belonging). On disclosing this Rebecca becomes tearful and says they do not like her because she is ugly and stupid (self-esteem). Love and belonging and self-esteem are said to be deficiency drives according to Maslow, and if these needs are not fulfilled a person may become ill.

Once the need is identified, you and Karen speak to Rebecca's school to identify ways in which Rebecca can become more included in activities and feel she belongs. Karen also discusses with Rebecca out-of-school activities she may enjoy.

Whilst this example demonstrates how a nurse could utilise the knowledge of Maslow's motivational theory to assist patients, the same understanding can help nurses develop their own well-being.

Motivation and locus of control

Rotter, and many others since, have considered the perceived locus of control – locus meaning where the control is situated or stems from. He suggested it has a big impact on behavioural motivation, especially health behaviours.

Rotter (1966)

Rotter suggested that the personality characteristic that influences a person's behaviour is whether they have a perception of internal or external control (locus of control). A person with an internal locus of control would believe they are in control of their behaviour, health and lifestyle, and that the main thing that affects their life is what they do themselves.

A person with an external locus of control would believe that the government, their parents or the university controls their behaviour. They may also suggest it is all down to chance and no one has control over them or anything else.

Activity

Given the following scenario would you say John, Joe and Jane have an internal or external locus of control and which is going to best facilitate their passing next time?

John, Joe and Jane have been studying hard for their nursing exams. They attended all the teaching sessions but the revision session had to be cancelled due to the teacher being ill. The teacher did leave some revision suggestions and handouts.

Jane went to bed early the night before the exam after a warm drink and a bath. She woke early the next morning and had a good breakfast.

John went to the pub with friends and had a few beers, arrived home and 'crashed out'; he found getting up the next morning difficult.

Joe spent the evening doing some last minute revision; he went to bed late and woke early.

Continued

> *All three students failed their exams but their responses were different:*
>
> John's response to his failure was, 'Well, that's life. They'll let me re-sit it and maybe I'll pass next time. It's a bit of a pain but I've never been lucky.'
> Joe's response was, 'I didn't do enough work, I should have started my revision earlier and tried harder. Next time I'll ask for a tutorial and organise myself better.'
> Jane's response was, 'If that teacher had turned up for our revision session I would have passed the exam; the teachers did not do their job properly. How do they expect us to pass under these circumstances?'

Response to activity

It has been said that people like Joe, who has an internal locus of control, would have better outcomes, including health, owing to their taking control and acting on information. Whereas Jane's and John's external locus of control could be considered problematic as they may not put into action healthy behaviours because they believe that other people or chance are in control, and not them.

This could be debatable as in Jane and John's situation their stress level may be low in response to their failure as they do not feel they are at fault, whereas Joe believes his success is dependent on his behaviour, which may increase his stress in the run-up to the re-sit exams.

Summary

So far we have considered a biological, psychodynamic and humanistic view of motivation, and the locus of control. We have moved through a process of the person having no conscious control over their motivation through to having control and then perception of control. It is suggested that to be emotionally intelligent, nurses need to manage their motivations. Therefore nurses who have good awareness of their own motivations and believe they have control over them, are in a better position to help others.

Social learning theory

Social learning theory offers two sets of motivator, both of which have been developed through modelling: intrinsic and extrinsic.

- *Intrinsic.* Motivation and its fulfilment come from within the person. It is where the person gains rewards for their behaviour from within themselves, such as assisting with a patient's personal hygiene leaving the nurse with a feeling of pleasure.
- *Extrinsic.* Motivation to enact a behaviour comes from outside the person. For a nurse this could be where the person being cared for would like to leave the unit and the nurse offers to escort them, to be recognised by her mentor as being caring, or when a nurse knows that if she does not respond rapidly to a call she will be punished.

Deci et al. (1991, cited Sternberg 2000) offered some suggestions that might be useful for nurse managers on how to facilitate a change from external to internal motivation in the nursing team:

- Enable the nurse to feel competent and socially related to others.
- Offer choices for implementing the desired behaviour.
- Avoid threats.
- Avoid tangible rewards (e.g. money); using praise does less damage to intrinsic motivation.
- If rewards are to be given, use them as surprises or extras.
- Recognise how the nurse feels about a given behaviour or task, whether negative or positive.
- Show the nurse that their knowledge and skills are recognised and that they are competent and autonomous.
- Do not use words such as *should, ought* or *must.*

Section summary

The psychological theories that have been considered have suggested that nurses can be motivated by their biological, psychological and social needs. Nurses can be taught to be self-motivating and have a perception of their own control, which may be considered preferable.

Perception

There are two distinct areas of study in perception: the sensational perception (derived from the senses), which mainly deals with objects (usually known as object perception), and social perception, in regard to people (person perception).

There are some features that both object and people perception have in common:

- Selection – focusing on a particular object or part of a person's behaviour
- Organisation – trying to gain an understanding of the complete object or person
- Inference – making assumptions about the object or person that there is no specific evidence for at the moment of perception.

Object perception

There are a number of psychological theories about how people perceive objects and why they get it wrong at times. These have developed out of the cognitive perspective, and cognitive researchers have tried to understand how information from the senses is received, processed, stored and retrieved. There are four major approaches to this:

- Bottom up
- Top down
- Cyclic
- Gestalt

Bottom up

This theory was developed by Gibson (1966) and is called the theory of direct perception. His research was mainly in the area of visual perception and he suggested that there was no need for inferences because there was enough unambiguous information in the environment for people to perceive an object.

Top down

Gregory (1966), who suggested that perceptions are unconscious inferences, developed a constructivist theory. He thought that people already have an idea of what objects they are going to find in their mind; they then check the environment for these objects. This is called a perceptual hypothesis and can lead to illusions when a person finds what they expect rather than what is there. He also suggested that people look for perceptual constancy; an example of a perceptual constancy is that if something is further away it is smaller.

There are similarities between Gibson's and Gregory's theories (Gross 1996, p. 216):

- Visual perception is mediated by light reflected from surfaces and objects.
- Some kind of physiological system is needed to perceive.
- Perception is an active process.
- Perceptual experiences can be influenced by learning.

Differences between Gibson's and Gregory's theories are (Gross 1996):

- The nature of learning is different.
- Gregory's learning involves construction or synthesis
- Gibson's learning involved analysis.

Cyclic

Neisser's (1976) cyclic model of perception offered a process where the mind was actively searching for information from the environment and the environment was providing rich information to be analysed. Therefore this model involves both bottom up and top down theories.

Box 2.1 Example demonstrating three theories of object perception

In the clinical skills laboratories at the university you and one of your peers, Kate, have been asked to put together a 'giving set' to intravenously give a patient fluids. You both have all the equipment set out on a trolley. Kate quickly assembles her set but you slowly and methodically identify which pieces join together. You both achieve the task and afterwards you ask Kate how she completed the task so quickly. Kate said that when she had been on her clinical placement she had seen a giving set hanging from a drip stand. Kate had used her previous experience to guide her in the task (top down) and had pieced together the set (bottom up). She had used both theories of perception leading to a cyclical approach, whereas you had no previous experience and so had methodically pieced together each small part (bottom up).

Gestalt

Whereas Gregory's theory focused on *inferences* (ideas or hypotheses) and Gibson's theory on information from the *selected* object (focus on the detail), the gestalt approach focuses on *organisation*. The gestalt theorists suggested that people focused on wholes rather than isolated sensations. They offered a number of laws by which people adopted a best-fit approach to perception (see Figure 2.1):

- Proximity – if items are close together they are seen as a whole
- Similarity – things that are similar to each other are grouped together
- Continuity – people tend to look for continuity of items rather than separate items
- Closure – when parts of what appears to be an object are missing they are not noticed
- Part–whole relationships – sense will be made of an overall picture rather than sense being made of the smaller parts

Illusions

There are illusions to be found in all of the senses but most talked about are visual illusions and these fall into four types:

- Distortions – misperceive (examples: Muller-Lyer, Ponzo, Titchner, etc)
- Ambiguous figures – same input different perceptions (examples: Rubin vase, Leeper's woman)
- Paradoxical figures – false assumptions (examples: Penrose impossible objects, Escher's pictures)
- Fictions – see what is not there (example: Kanizsa triangle)

Illusions are difficult to explain unless there is a mental processing part of perception.

Summary

Although it is important for nurses to be aware of object perception theories, particularly in the area of illusions, they may offer little information on who should be a nurse. However, they do offer an explanation of how a nurse may perceive the world and why there may be individual differences in perception. This recognition of differing perceptions and of illusions can be useful for nurses and can aid them in their interventions with patients or clients.

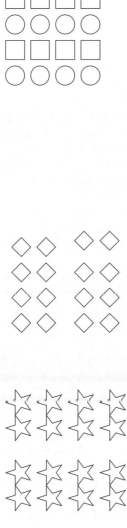

Proximity – stars appear to be in columns whereas diamonds appear to be in rows due to proximity of the shapes

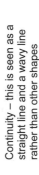

Similarity – similar shapes are grouped together; despite proximity the circles and squares are seen as separate columns

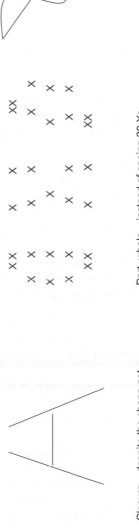

Part–whole – instead of seeing 29 Xs people see oxo

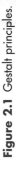

Continuity – this is seen as a straight line and a wavy line rather than other shapes

Closure – despite the shape not being complete it will usually be seen as an A

Figure 2.1 Gestalt principles.

Social perception

In social perception as well as cognitive perceptual illusions what we 'see' might not always be correct.

Rungapadiachy (1999) argues that in social perception we do not always see accurately what someone is really thinking or feeling; in fact he says that sometimes people, for a variety of reasons, want us 'to perceive what is in fact not true'.

Cognitive perspective within social perception

There are four models of the thinking person within social perception:

- Consistency seekers – where the person seeks to reduce inconsistencies in thoughts about the social world as inconsistency causes dissonance or psychological discomfort for the individual.
- Naïve scientist – where people try to understand other people by generating inferences or hypotheses like scientists; this is the area within which the attribution theories developed.
- Cognitive miser – developed in response to the naïve scientist as it was found people had limited processing capacity and so found short-cuts to understanding others, using heuristics or rules of thumb.
- Motivated tactician – developed from the cognitive miser model and in response to the consistency model, it acknowledges the role of emotion and motivation in perception.

Attribution theories

The correspondent theory

Attribution theories accept the person as a naïve scientist, and that they are a logical, rational, thinking being. Jones and Davis (1965, cited Hogg & Vaughan 1998) developed an attribution theory called the correspondent theory. They suggest that people make correspondent inferences. This is where an observed behaviour closely relates to a personality trait – they correspond. Inferences about people's behaviour are based on the disposition of the person (their personality/traits) and intentionality (that behaviour exhibited gained the intended response). The disposition of the person is assessed by the distinction between one choice of behaviour and another.

Other influences on the assessment of disposition are:

- Choice
- Social desirability
- Roles
- Prior expectations

Box 2.2   Example of the correspondent theory of attribution

You observe one of the nurses offering to make a person a drink as they have been waiting for some time for test results. The nurse could be said to be kind and considerate. This is a correspondent attribute because both the behaviour and the attributed disposition (kind and considerate) are similar.

This would be further weighed up by judging whether the nurse had had any choice in their behaviour, whether offering a drink was part of their role, whether you would have expected them to do this and whether it could be seen as a socially desirable behaviour.

If the nurse in charge had told the nurse to offer the person a drink, the disposition of kindness would not be attributed because the behaviour was not seen to have intentionality and there would be little choice.

Kelley's covariance model

Kelley's covariance model (1967, cited Davey 2004) refers to the dispositional characteristics a person is seen to have when something is known of the person and of the social norms for the particular behaviour. The decisions made about dispositions are based on:

- Consensus – would other people behave in the same way?
- Distinctiveness – is this something the person only does in certain circumstances?
- Consistency – how often does the person exhibit this behaviour?

Box 2.3   Example of covariance model, part 1

The nurse always arrives early and is well prepared at the beginning of their duty to provide care.

- Consensus – some other nurses would do this but not all of them – consensus is low.
- Distinctiveness – this is something that the nurse does every shift – distinctiveness is low.
- Consistency – the nurse always does this so it is consistent – consistency is high.

Kelley suggests that if consensus is low and distinctiveness is low but consistency is high, the causal attribution is to the actor, in this case the nurse. In other words, if the behaviour is something that is done just by this nurse consistently, it is attributed to the nurse's disposition.

Box 2.4 Part 2

The behaviour would be attributed to the nurse's disposition – the nurse is perhaps an organised person.

If it something that is done by lots of people (consensus high) in this situation (distinctiveness high) and only in this situation (consistency low), then circumstances would be the causal attribution or a situational reason.

Box 2.5 Part 3

If all nurses arrived early and were well prepared, the causal attribution could be to the circumstances – at the beginning of a shift of duty nurses are prepared.

How are others perceived?

Attribution theory offers one explanation of how others are seen. It explains how inferences are made about people's behaviour, leading to perception of dispositional characteristics through certain rules, but there are other theories of how others are perceived.

Implicit personality theories are used, or clusters of traits. These can offer short-cuts when there is little information available to make an accurate assessment. Some of these methods are:

- The halo effect
- Stereotyping
- Importance of names
- Importance of physical appearance

Asch, in 1946, conducted a study demonstrating the importance of two key dispositional characteristics – warm and cold. He called this the *halo effect*. If someone was labelled warm, a number of other characteristics were attributed to them – the positive halo. If someone had been labelled cold regardless of other characteristics, they gained a negative halo and led to other negative characteristics being attributed to them.

Names and *physical appearance* also generated a consistent group of characteristics. If a person is fat they are considered jolly; if they have eyes close together they are considered untrustworthy. Certain names are ascribed to certain personality types; for example, Matthew is seen in a more positive light than Wayne.

These could be considered stereotypes, but usually this term is reserved for whole social groups rather than individuals. There have been lengthy discussions on the usefulness of stereotypes as they can lead to discrimination, but some suggest they are a normal cognitive function, as are other implicit personality theories, to allow people to function when little information is available.

Case study   Demonstrating the halo effect

Jemma is a student nurse on a busy ward. There are two deputy charge nurses on the ward; one named Maria is described as warm by previous students, and the other, Janine, is described as cold by previous students. When Jemma is feeling insecure in her ability to help a patient she approaches Maria and seeks support, whereas when Jemma is faced with an aggressive patient she approaches Janine for support. Both Maria and Janine give Jemma support with the situation, but the halo effect continues as Jemma has requested support in a manner that supports the halo.

How do we influence how others perceive us?

For all nurses there is the expectation that whatever their personality type, they are seen to behave in a professional manner. Therefore it is important that nurses are aware of how they can influence how others perceive them. Others' perceptions are influenced in a number of ways:

- Impression management
- Self-presentation
- Consistency
- Self-monitoring
- Self-disclosure

Impression management and self-presentation involve a certain level of emotional intelligence in that techniques used in impression management can only be developed with *self-awareness* and an understanding of how the individual is seen by others, which can be termed *empathy*. Once this is achieved the need is to *self-regulate* and use *social skills*. Techniques used to achieve impression management include behaviour matching, appreciating and flattering others. Demonstrating internal consistency is also important.

Self-monitors again manage their behaviour, as do the impression managers, by coming alongside others and 'being' what others need/ require/expect of them. Although low self-monitors could be considered lacking in social skills, they could be considered to have greater personal integrity because they hold to their views and beliefs and do not adjust these for the sake of others.

Case study   Simon's self-monitoring

Simon has worked for a number of years managing a small business, but felt himself drawn to mental health nursing. He has started the mental health nursing course and in his communication skills sessions he has become aware that he is inclined to talk over other people and to try force his opinion on them.

This awareness has allowed Simon to develop his communication skills, including self-regulation and social skills, and improve how others view him.

Self-disclosure partly determines how other people see us and there has been debate within nursing as to whether nurses should disclose information about themselves to the people they are caring for. The usual factors influencing self-disclosure in personal relationships, such as reciprocity, trust, quality of the relationship and gender, influencing self-disclosure within families and friendships, may not apply to professional relationships (see Chapter 6).

Section summary

This section has considered the psychological theories related to perception of objects and people and examined how useful the individual differences in perception are in understanding who should be a nurse as well as how to be a nurse. Key elements of social perception in this exploration are areas such as stereotypes, self-presentation, self-monitoring and self-disclosure, and these have been considered in relation to their suitability in nurses.

Chapter summary

Whilst nursing literature such as the NHS careers information suggests that all personality types are suitable candidates for nursing, an exploration of the research from a psychological approach would indicate that there are some boundaries. There are a number of personality theories that are helpful in our understanding of why a person may have the personality they do, but it is the individual differences within these personalities that are more useful for discriminating the personality needs of nursing. Both a cognitive rational intelligence and emotional intelligence were seen as necessary for nurses working within healthcare in our present society. This emotional intelligence seems to underpin both the motivational and perceptual requirements of nursing.

References

Bandura A. (1965) Influence of model's reinforcement contingencies on the acquisition of imitative responses. *Journal of Personality & Psychology*, 1, 589–595.

Cadman C. & Brewer J. (2001) Emotional intelligence: a vital prerequisite for recruitment in nursing. *Journal of Nursing Management*, 9, 321–324.

Davey G. (ed.) (2004) *Complete Psychology*. London: Hodder & Stoughton.

Fealy G.M. (2004) 'The good nurse': visions and values in images of the nurse. *Journal of Advanced Nursing*, 46(6), 649–656.

Freshwater D. & Stickley T. (2004) The heart of the art: emotional intelligence in nurse education. *Nursing Inquiry*, 11(2): 91–98.

Gardner H. (1983) *Frames of Mind: The Multiple Intelligence*. New York: Basic Books.

Gardner H. (1993) *Multiple Intelligence: The Theory in Practice*. New York: Basic Books.

Gardner H. (1999) Are there additional intelligence's? The case for naturalist, spiritual and existential intelligence's in J. Kane (ed.) *Education, Information and Transformation*. Englewood Cliffs, N.J.: Prentice Hall.

Gibson J.J. (1966) *The Senses Considered as Perceptual Systems*. Boston: Houghton Mifflin.

Goffman E. (1971) *The Presentation of Self in Everyday Life*. Harmondsworth: Penguin

Goleman D. (1995) *Emotional Intelligence*. New York: Bantam Books.

Green S. (1994) *Principles of Biopsychology*. Hove: Psychology Press, Taylor and Francis Group.

Gregory R.L. (1966) *Eye and Brain*. London: Weidenfeld & Nicholson.

Gross R. (1996) *Psychology: The Science of Mind and Behaviour*, 3rd edition. London: Hodder & Stoughton.

Gross R. (2001) *Psychology: The Science of Mind and Behaviour*, 4th edition. London: Hodder & Stoughton.

Malim T. & Birch A. (1998) *Introductory Psychology*. London: Macmillan Press.

Mayer J.D. & Salovey P. (1997) What is emotional intelligence? In Salovey P. & Mayer (eds.) *Emotional Development and Emotional Intelligence*, pp. 3–31. New York: Basic Books.

Neisser U. (1976) *Cognition and Reality*. San Fransisco, CA: W.H. Freeman.

NHS Careers (2005) Nursing and midwifery in the NHS, join the team and make a difference. Bristol: NHS Careers, and can be accessed at www.nhs.uk/careers.

Rotter J. (1966) Generalised expectancies for internal versus extenal control of reinforcement. *Psychological Monographs*, 30(1), 1–26.

Rungapadiachy Dev. M. (1999) *Interpersonal Communication and Psychology for Health Care Professionals, Theory and Practice*. Oxford: Butterworth Heinemann.

Sternberg R.J. (2000) *Pathways to Psychology*, 2nd edition. London: Harcourt Brace.

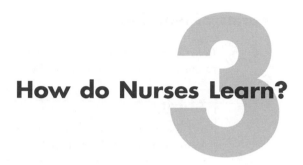

How do Nurses Learn?

Learning Objectives

It is generally recognised that all people need to learn throughout their lives, although a number of people believe that nursing is a vocation rather than learnt skills and knowledge. This chapter considers the importance of learning for nurses and the people that they care for. The learning objectives are:

- Discuss the importance of learning from each of the given psychological perspectives.
- Identify what 'learning people skills' is and how this is relevant to nursing care.
- Explore how an understanding of learning supports health promotion activities.
- Describe the relationship between learning and the uptake of treatment.

Introduction

This chapter focuses on nurses learning through pre-registration programmes, including the use of role models such as mentors and consultant nurses. It considers the importance of different learning theories and then goes on to consider how an understanding of learning can facilitate the nursing activity of health promotion.

Theories of learning

Learning is defined as 'a long lasting change in behaviour based on experience, or adaptation to the environment' (Papalia et al. 1998).

Activity

Why is it important to understand how nurses learn?
What might influence this learning?

Response to activity

It is important to understand how nurses learn at university and on their practice placements. The lecturers, practice educators and individual nurses need to identify factors which enhance the nurse's ability to learn how to provide quality care for the people with whom they work. If this understanding is developed together, the educators and the individual nurses can promote the learning process and achieve their goal of high quality evidence-based care.

It is also important for nurses to understand how they learn as it can, in turn, aid their understanding of how the people with whom they work may be helped to learn about their health difficulties and the care they need. This can include everyday life-skills such as self-care skills, including self-medication, specific rehabilitation and coping strategies.

Some nurses and the people that they work with may have specific learning disabilities. It is important to understand these learning disabilities and what can be done to help overcome or cope with them. There is a broad spectrum of learning disability, from people who need guidance on note-taking to people who need assistance with all areas of living.

Understanding how learning can be affected by illness and disease, or vice versa, how illness and disease can be affected by the person's ability to learn, should also be part of a nurse's repertoire.

Box 3.1   Relationship between health and learning

Illness or disease affecting learning:
A person who is suffering from dementia may have problems with learning how to use an electrical device such as a new cooker.

Ability to learn affecting illness or disease:
A person with diabetes who has a learning disability may have problems with adhering to the treatment regime, which could have negative consequences for their health.

Learning is considered to be one of the fundamental living skills and psychologists offer some explanations for how people, including nurses, do this. The behaviourists suggest that all a person is, their personality, behaviours, attitudes, etc. are learnt (see Chapter 1).

The behavioural psychologists

Introduction

The early behaviourists offered two basic forms of learning, which they called classical and operant conditioning. These theories, though, were preceded by the concept of habituation, which is seen in the most primitive organisms – learning occurs through familiarisation. Familiarisation allows the creature to recognise that the stimulus is not harmful and so the organism ignores its presence. These theories of learning were later developed by Bandura to include social learning theory.

Classical conditioning

Classical conditioning is the label given to learning through the Pavlovian stimulus–response theory of learning. The conditioning or learning occurs when a person reflexively responds to a given stimulus. This reflexive response can be trained (conditioned) to occur with other stimuli that do not provoke this response, by a process of association. A reflexive response is gained from a previously unassociated stimulus. Hence this can be referred to as learning by association; if one stimulus is associated with another stimulus that produces a certain response, after a period of time both stimuli will gain the same response.

Case study   Impact of classical conditioning on Alexa's learning

When Alexia, a student nurse, was feeling anxious about her abilities, she spoke to her mentor. The mentor sat down with Alexia, made her a hot drink, listened to her concerns and talked to her about the things she did well (unconditioned stimulus). Alexia, after each of these sessions, went away aware of her abilities and having confidence (unconditioned response) to undertake her nursing role. This happened for the whole of Alexia's placement in that area. In the next placement, when she felt anxious she made herself a hot drink (conditioned stimulus) and afterwards she felt the confidence (conditioned response) of the previous situation. Alexia had associated the hot drink with the feeling of confidence.

Operant conditioning

Learning also occurs in a more explicit manner, where a person will learn that to do one thing rather than another produces a reward (operant conditioning). Skinner developed this theory of learning and it can be observed in many animals as well as people. Skinner suggested that in the real world animals do not respond to just one stimulus at a time, so he explored how they *operated* within their environments with multiple stimuli.

In the case of operant conditioning, learning is either in the form of training by a teacher or a matter of 'trial and error'; in either situation rewards or punishment influence the learning.

Case study   Simba's care develops through operant conditioning

Simba, a first-year student nurse, is given the task of assisting Janet, a person he is caring for, to eat her meal. Janet is unable to talk. Simba has been told Janet cannot feed herself and he observes she cannot pick up her cutlery. Janet was obviously unhappy when Simba offered to feed her. Initially Simba picked the cutlery up and tried to place them in Janet's hands. Janet could hold the cutlery but her hands and arms were not strong enough or co-ordinated enough to cut or pick up the food. Simba then tried to assist by holding Janet's hands to give strength and co-ordination; while this was effective Janet still did not appear happy with this arrangement. After a little time Simba put the soup into a mug that Janet could pick up and hold in two hands, which gave strength and helped with the co-ordination. Simba then put the meat between pieces of bread and put it in her hand. Janet appeared extremely pleased. Through this process of trial and error Simba had learnt how to assist Janet and had managed to gain the reward of improving the emotional well-being of Janet.

Social learning theory

Another form of learning that builds on classical and operant conditioning is social learning theory. This theory was developed by Bandura and acknowledged a cognitive element to learning. The theory suggests that learning can occur not only by association and reward but also by observing others' behaviour and imitating it – *vicarious learning*.

> **Box 3.2   Example of vicarious learning**
>
> Nurses are required to be able to offer cardio-pulmonary resuscitation, which students are taught in the clinical skills laboratory. The students observed how the clinical demonstrator carried out the procedure of cardio-pulmonary resuscitation (*observe*) and then they copied the behaviour (*imitate*).

Albert Bandura (1977) and colleagues developed this theory of social learning through a number of experiments which demonstrated that observational or vicarious learning could occur. For this type of learning to take place there needs to be another person or people to learn from; this person is usually referred to as the *role model*. There are three cognitive components that influence the likelihood of learning from a role model. These are:

- Attention
- Memory
- Motivation

Effective role models

There are certain features that make a role model effective; these features enhance the vicarious learning. An effective role model possesses the following attributes:

- They are rewarded.
- They are similar enough to imitate.
- They are well thought of or respected socially.

Bandura also identified that, along with the concrete skills of the example given, people, especially children, also develop their values and attitudes, along with problem solving and self-evaluation, from their social environment.

Nursing role models

Role modelling can clearly be seen in nurse education; nurses, like other students, are given personal tutors but they also have mentors in the care environments. Both personal tutors and mentors can become role models, but the mentor in the practice area fulfils this role more effectively as they are putting knowledge and skills into effect. Student nurses can be seen to learn not only nursing skills, such as how to monitors a person's blood pressure, through vicarious learning but also what is understood by professional behaviour and how to respond to suffering experienced in those they care for.

Nursing students spend half their education in the care environment and so the nurse mentors spend a lot of time with them. Student nurses during their course have to demonstrate not only academic ability but also clinical competence. These competencies are set by the NMC, the professional body for nurses, and are presented to students to achieve in four domains: Professional and Ethical Practice, Care Delivery, Care Management, Personal and Professional Development.

The student nurse needs to demonstrate to their clinical assessor, who may be their mentor as well, that they are competent in each of the areas, which involve all the abilities identified within social learning theory: concrete skills, problem solving, attitudes, values and self-evaluation. The main way in which nurses learn these attributes in the care environment is through their role model. These care behaviours are monitored by the mentor who offers reinforcement or reward in the form of feedback on achievement.

Case study   Role modelling facilitates Precious's learning

Precious is a second-year student nurse, undertaking her first community-based placement. George is her mentor. He will support Precious by initially taking her with him on visits and he will take the lead, but by the end of her placement George expects that Precious will take the lead on the visits (role modelling).

Precious watches George and how he introduces them to the clients; she notices his respectful manner in the clients' houses and how he gives them time to explain what has been happening to them and what their concerns are. When Precious and George return to their base unit he shows Precious how he documents the visit and explains where he gained the evidence for his interventions. At the end of her placements Precious is able to introduce herself and George in a professional respectful manner, conduct the interview with the clients, document their interactions and explain to George what evidence base she had used to support her interventions.

Through role modelling Precious has learnt a number of professional skills, ranging from concrete to attitudinal, and the value of basing her professional practice on evidence.

Self-efficacy

Self-efficacy is a person's belief in their ability to achieve something and is an important factor in prompting behaviour or motivation. The social learning theory approach suggests that a person's motivation to attempt modelling behaviour is dependent on the person believing they can accomplish that behaviour. Self-efficacy is learnt from previous experiences of the same or similar situation and the feedback gained. It is important that nurses are aware of and develop their own self-efficacy and that of the people with whom they work, to achieve positive outcomes.

Using behavioural theory to maximise learning

Student nurses can use the theories described to enhance their ability to learn in a number of ways. Using the behavioural theory of Skinner (1938, cited in Child 1997) the following would enhance learning:

- They should break the learning into small steps or chunks building on previous learning.
- Initially they should reward themselves immediately and on every occasion, but this should reduce to intermittent rewards after the learning has been established.
- Feedback should be sought promptly, with each step small enough to be achievable; motivation for the goal and learning are increased.
- They should seek and identify the best method of achievement of the desired learning.

Summary

The behaviourists offer nurses understanding of their own learning and the learning of the patients or clients with whom they work. This understanding can enhance nurses' ability to develop their own learning and facilitate the learning of others. The key components of the behavioural approach to learning are association, reinforcement (reward) and observation and imitation. Importantly, the behaviourists do not make any distinctions between those considered more able and less able to learn the learning approaches. Therefore if the nurse has a learning disability, or their patients or clients do, these learning theories still apply.

The cognitive psychologists

Introduction

The cognitive perspective can be seen as an extension of the behaviourist perspective in that there is an acceptance that behaviour is
learnt and that in any situation there is a stimulus and a response.
The cognitive psychologists seek to understand what happens between
stimulus and response, because they recognise that there is not
always a predictable automatic response to any given stimulus (see
Chapter 1).

They recognise that student nurses do not passively accept knowledge but are active recipients making an effort to understand and
retain it. The nurse teacher's role is to facilitate the nurse's discovery
of knowledge. It is suggested by those who adopt the schema theory
(a cognitive theory of thought organisation) of cognition that nurses
need to be prepared prior to attending a teaching session, perhaps by
set reading, so that they can incorporate their new understanding to
previously structured schemas.

The theory is similar to the behaviourists' approach in that there is
a recognised need for information to be separated into small achievable
chunks or sub-goals, to reach understanding of the area. Feedback on
the development of the nurse's learning is crucial as this becomes part
of the learning and allows them to move on to the next chunk with
confidence and increased understanding.

The cognitive psychologists are particularly interested in thoughts,
memory, motivation, attention, perception and intelligence. Each of
these topics can be seen as influential in learning.

Intelligence

Whilst intelligence has long been thought to be a key factor in learning,
and despite there being numerous intelligence testing scales available,
identifying what intelligence is and how this relates to achievements
is debatable (see Chapter 2). The behaviourists suggest that all people
access the same processes to learn, regardless of starting point, but the
cognitive psychologists are interested in what intelligence is, how it
can be measured and the impact it has on human functioning. As seen
in Chapter 2 there are a number of definitions of intelligence, with
Gardener proposing multiple intelligence.

Whilst problematic, intelligence tests such as the Wechsler intelligence test, and those which test specific areas linked to intelligence (i.e.
spatial ability), continue to be popular, particularly in education, as
they are fairly good at predicting academic success (Anderson 2000).

This would therefore suggest that intelligence may be linked to learning, at least academically.

Motivation, attention and perception

Cognitive psychologists suggest that motivation, attention and perception are all linked to learning. Motivation and attention are specifically identified in social learning theory, which forms a link between behavioural and cognitive approaches to learning. For learning to occur, it is generally assumed that the item needs to be accurately perceived; faulty learning can occur if the person misperceives an item.

Case study   The impact of perception on Mai-Ling's learning

Mai-Ling is an adult branch student nurse. The teaching session on her programme today is psychological approaches to communication. Mai-Ling discusses this with the other students prior to the session and their perception is that the lecturer taking the session is a mental health lecturer and that the focus of the session is different ways of talking to people with mental health problems (perception). She sits in the teaching room but does not give the session her full attention as she believes it is not relevant to her. Her motivation to participate in the activities is low and she leaves the session believing she has learnt nothing.

If Mai-Ling and the other students had believed the focus of the session was to assist them to communicate with people who had different health problems, maybe from their present area of practice (perception), this may have led them to give the session more attention and to have more motivation to participate and increase their learning opportunity.

Memory

Memory and learning appear to be inextricably linked. Learning cannot occur unless the person has the capacity to retain and retrieve the skill, information or attitude. Most learning approaches aim to increase long-term memory or deep learning. Anderson (2000) identifies that practice or repetition is the power law of learning and improves memory. Factors that affect memory will also have an impact on learning. This is particularly important for nurses as they are frequently attempting to learn new things or teach things to patients when they are under stress. Memory can be damaged through illness and disease and interfered with by processes such as stress.

Factors influencing learning

Factors that influence learning can be divided into external or environmental and internal:

- Environmental factors influencing learning: noise, temperature, resources available, etc.
- Internal factors influencing learning: intelligence, motivation, perception, attention, memory, previous learning.

Box 3.3   Examples of what might influence learning

Reduced opportunity for learning could occur in this situation:
External: It is a warm afternoon and the lecturer has chosen to use the projector to display the teaching materials. As the sun is shining the blinds have been closed to enhance the definition of the projected image. In the darkened room the windows are open due to the warm, stuffy atmosphere. The noise of the traffic on the road outside is a continuous rumble, which obscures the lecturer's voice.
Internal: The student nurse had been to a nightclub the night before and is feeling very tired. Due to the exertion of the night before and getting up late they rushed to the university and did not have breakfast, so at lunchtime ate more than usual.

Increased opportunity for learning could occur in this situation:
External: The teaching takes place in an air-conditioned teaching room with visual aids on the walls and shelves. The lecturer uses a variety of teaching resources, with student nurses moving from one resource to another in small groups. The lecturer spends short periods of time talking and the student nurses interactively discuss what has been said. The students are given the opportunity to practise and repeat the material.
Internal: The student nurse is aware of the topic being taught the next day and so has read the notes provided by the lecturer. They get up early enough to have breakfast and have a steady journey to the teaching session. They recognise the importance of the topic for their learning and focus on the discussions, and actively take part.

Cognitive theories suggest that the nurse needs to be an active participant in the process to develop learning; the responsibility for this lies with both teacher and learner. These theories would suggest that to maximise learning the following is useful (Reece & Walker 1997):

- Take full advantage of the structure of the subject and make clear links between the subject and previously learnt material.
- Nurse teachers should offer preparatory information so the nurses are primed for the learning experience.
- Nurses need to make their own links with previous learning and experiences, particularly personal ones encouraged by their teachers.
- Plan teaching material so the nurses discover new knowledge themselves.
- Use specific clearly-linked questioning.
- Nurses should discuss their new understandings (opportunity for repetition).

Gagne (1970) developed a hierarchy of primitive learning from habituation (identified by the behaviourists) through to complex problem solving (explored by the cognitive psychologists):

- Habituation – familiarisation
- Classical conditioning – association of stimulus and response – involuntary behaviour
- Operant conditioning – stimulus, response, reward – voluntary behaviour which is needs led
- Chaining – two or more stimulus response behaviours linked together – sequencing behaviour
- Verbal association – sequencing of verbal behaviours
- Discrimination learning – more than one behavioural response to same stimulus
- Concept learning – using cognitive skills (memory, classification) to recognise similarity of stimuli, leading to similar behaviour responses but also involving discrimination
- Rule learning – behaviour involving two or more concepts
- Problem solving – the manipulation rules and making new rules to achieve goals

Summary

Cognitive psychologists recognise that learning is an important process strongly linked to memory, which has a direct impact on other cognitive activities such as language acquisition, problem solving and motivation.

This approach focuses on the roles of student nurses and nurse teachers; both have important roles in the process of learning. The student needs to make efforts to learn and the teacher need to ensure the 'to be learnt' material is presented and worked on in an appropriate manner.

Humanistic psychologists

Introduction

The humanistic movement started in the 1950s in response to the mechanistic approach taken by the behaviourists and the conflict and distress focused on by the psychodynamic psychologists. They accepted that learning was important and they also acknowledged the importance of innate potential and unconscious processes. Despite this their focus was much more optimistic, identifying the person as an individual whole being with unique potential. They suggested that all people are moving towards self-actualisation, to achieve their potential (see Chapters 1 and 6).

Humanistic approaches to learning recognise the unique potential of each learner and their individual learning styles. They see each person as able to identify their own learning needs as they move towards self-actualisation. The teacher or educator is seen more as a facilitator rather than a giver of information or behaviour modifier. The facilitator works with the student as equal participants; they behave towards each other as equal adults. The humanistic approach has been captured in adult learning approaches.

Case study   Enquiry-based learning

A group of student nurses are given a scenario of a client or patient in pain. They are offered some lectures on the physiology and psychology of pain, which they can attend along with guided study on their particular care group, nursing assessments and interventions. The student nurses also have regular sessions organised with a facilitator. The facilitator accesses the approach outlined by Rogers as necessary for a therapeutic relationship, treating the students with respect and unconditional positive regard. The student nurses are expected to organise their own time, collect information and develop understanding of the client or patient and their care needs. This can be labelled, in learning terms, as self-directed learning, enquiry-based learning or problem-based learning.

Humanistic approaches to teaching and learning are similar to those of the cognitive approaches but they are less structured by the teacher, and the students are facilitated to structure their learning in the most appropriate ways for themselves.

This approach emphasises:

- Personality drives
- Growth towards autonomy and competence
- The innate motivation towards self-actualisation and the growth of the individual
- Active search for meaning
- Individual personal goals
- Attention to the social setting within which the students are learning

Nurses can use this approach to develop their teaching and learning by (Reece & Walker 1997):

- Facilitating choice within the learning environment
- Establishing a warm, positive atmosphere
- Facilitating, encouraging, helping the learning process
- Encouraging positive feeling of all members of the teaching environment
- Using experiential learning and role play
- Considering the effect, habits and attitudes within the learning environment

Learning people skills

'The emphasis in nursing in recent years has been on tailoring care to meet the needs of the patient or client. If we are to understand the needs of others, we need to understand our own needs.' (Burnard 2000, p. 4).

As Burnard says, the emphasis in healthcare is to be patient or client focused. This means that probably the most important skills that nurses need to learn are human skills or people skills. This links closely to the identification in Chapter 2 that nurses need to develop their emotional intelligence.

It is important that nurses understand their own needs and where these come from, and how they can attempt to achieve them. This is known as self-awareness. This is explored in Chapter 6 along with managing the therapeutic relationship, but this chapter is concerned with how nurses learn about themselves and others.

Burnard (2002, p. 58) recommends experiential and reflective approaches to learning human skills. He suggests the characteristics of experiential learning are:

- There is an emphasis on action.
- Students are encouraged to reflect on their practice.

- A clarifying approach is adopted by the facilitator.
- There is an accent on personal experience.
- Human experience is valued as a source of learning.

If these elements are compared to the psychological theories of learning already outlined, it can be seen that experiential learning incorporates both the humanistic and cognitive behavioural approaches. Experiential learning is essentially learning about people through interacting with them. The experiences of interacting with others can be linked to evidence-based practice, which is also expected of nurses in the current socio-political climate through the use of structured reflection. Johns (2000), along with a number of others, offers nurses a structured model of reflection, which facilitates this evidence-based practice.

Johns' (2000) model of reflection comprises:

- Phenomenon
  - Describe the experience
- Causal
  - What essential factors contributed to this experience?
- Context
  - What are the significant background factors to experience?
- Reflection
  - What was I trying to achieve?
  - Why did I intervene?
  - What were the consequences of my actions for (myself, the patient, the family)?
  - How did I feel about this experience?
  - How did the patient feel?
  - What factors, knowledge, influenced my decisions and action?
- Alternative actions
  - What other choices did I have?
  - What would be the consequences of these other choices?
- Learning
  - How do I now feel about this experience?
  - What have I learnt from this experience?

Structured reflection is expected to be undertaken by student nurses, both individually and in groups. This should not end when a nurse becomes registered, as a qualified nurse is expected by their professional body (NMC) to continue to develop throughout their career and one of the methods of doing this is through reflection. For registered nurses reflection can continue in a structured way through clinical supervision to ensure nursing care is maintained and developed.

Summary

Experiential learning is a core component of nurse education and learning the necessary people skills through clinical skills training in laboratories, reflective practice groups, assignments, and professional practice with clients or patients. It incorporates the elements of cognitive behavioural and humanistic approaches. It is eclectic but focused on the specific needs of the learner.

Psychodynamic psychologists

The psychodynamic approach does not offer nurses an explicit theory of learning but it does offer an understanding of what might interfere with a person's ability to learn.

The psychodynamic approach is concerned with how people learn the rules, attitudes and values from, initially, parents and significant others. Psychodynamic psychologists are interested in early relationships and how these influence the adult personality. They do not offer much guidance for how adult nurses might learn, other than through analysis to resolve underlying issues. Despite this, if a person has unresolved issues that have not been addressed, this will have an impact on their personality and ability to learn and develop. Anna Freud and Melanie Klein (psychodynamic theorists), who developed play therapy, recognised the importance of giving feedback or educating the child about their experiences so that they could continue to develop.

The psychodynamic therapists aim to help the person develop a full sense or understanding of themselves, where they can achieve their needs and desires within the social boundaries. To do this a person's ego must be able to balance the conflict between the id and superego and to have successfully negotiated the psychosexual stages (see Chapters 1, 2 and 6). If this cannot be managed, it will have an impact on the person's personality.

There is a lot of literature available that suggests there is a link between personality and health. Poor health or illness, in turn, can have an impact on a person's ability to learn.

Links between personality, health and illness may be due to the following (Morrison & Bennett 2006):

- Personality can be predictive of illness such as the link between type 'A' personality and cardiovascular disease.
- Personality may be perceived to change due to illness – thinking, affect and behavioural change due to chronic illness.
- Personality may promote behaviours linked to illness, such as alcohol abuse.

- Personality may play a role in illness progression due to unhelpful coping strategies.

Ill health can have profound impact on learning; a person acutely ill may experience pain and anxiety, both of which reduce concentration, attention and memory. Each of these is involved in learning, according to the cognitive and humanistic theorists.

Biological psychologists

The biological psychologists' approach to learning is focused on internal factors such as localisation of brain function, homeostasis, damage and neural readiness, and the external factors that influence these. Issues such as genetic predisposition, prenatal damage or disorder, and problems at birth and in the post-natal period, all can have a long-term effect on the baby/child/person's capacity for learning.

These problems may be due to illness, disease, trauma, malnutrition or even stress and lack of early stimulation. Even if there is no major damage or genetic abnormality, changes in hormones, neurotransmitters and blood sugar level can all have an impact on learning.

Case study   Ash explores the impact of biological functioning on learning

Ash has a placement with a school nurse. The school nurse is having a number of adolescents sent to her late morning with headaches, tiredness and lack of attention. These were having an impact on the pupils' ability to learn, while in the classroom and through leaving their lessons. The school nurse asked Ash to search through the nursing database to see if he could find any reasons or interventions that might address this problem. Ash found a study by Sweeney et al. in 2006 who found similar problems in an inner-city high school. Their approach had been to offer a 9am nutrition break; this reduced the midmorning hunger, inability to focus, tiredness and stomach-aches and increased the ability of the adolescents to learn.

Brain regions involved in learning and memory

The biopsychologists, along with cognitive psychologists, recognise that memory and learning are extremely difficult to study separately. They offer an understanding of the anatomy and physiology that underlie the learning described by the behaviourists, and work with cognitive psychologists to develop a clearer understanding of how the psychological processes identified by them can be explained in biological terms.

Many regions of the brain are involved with learning and memory, but biopsychologists are able to differentiate between those parts of the brain involved in what are labelled by cognitive psychologists as declarative and non-declarative memory or learning.

Declarative memory and learning
Declarative memory and learning consist of episodic information (stored in the cortex, probably right frontal and temporal regions) and semantic information (stored probably in the temporal lobes). Episodic memory and learning involve autobiographical information, where and when things happened, whereas semantic memory and learning involve general information such as the meaning of words.

Procedural or non-declarative memory and learning
This part of memory and learning relates to skills acquisition, priming (more likely to use a word recently heard) and conditioning that has been learnt but is not accessible for verbal explanation. Skills learning has been found to occur in the basal ganglia, motor cortex and cerebellum. Priming can be perceptual or conceptual and reduces activity in the occipital or frontal cortex, and the two types of conditioning occur either in the cerebellar circuit or hippocampus and cortex.

Localisation of brain activity
Despite the discrete areas described previously, learning may involve many areas of the brain, but the localisations offer a limited overview of the brain activity involved. Biopsychologists have found that emotions play an important part in memory and learning, both anatomically and physiologically. This is particularly important to nurses when they are explaining treatments and conditions to patients or clients, as they could be distressed at the time and find learning and memory for new information difficult.

Biopsychologists' understanding and explanations of learning and memory are useful to nurses as they can offer an explanation for their own learning and lack of ability to learn certain things, and for those they care for.

Box 3.4   Example of nurses working with a person with a learning and memory problem that has an organic cause

Nurses working in mental health, adult or learning disability services may come into contact with people with a diagnosis of Korsakoff's syndrome. This problem is exhibited by confusion, memory loss, inability to learn new information and confabulation. It is suggested that confabulation (making up events to fill in the gaps in memory) occurs because the person's intellect is not affected.

The problem occurs in people with long-term alcoholism; the brain damage leading to the exhibited behaviour is due to thiamine (vitamin B) deficiency. This nutritional deficiency leads to shrunken diseased mamillary bodies, damage to basal frontal lobes and damage to the dorsomedial thalamus.

People with this problem may be nursed by one of a number of branches, owing to the reason for the problem (addiction, nutritional deficiency and brain damage) exhibiting behaviour and care needs.

The condition can be treated with thiamine but this will only halt the progression of the problem, not rectify the damage. If the person had received thiamine at an early stage of addiction they would not have progressed to Korsakoff's syndrome.

Summary

The biological psychologists offer an anatomical and physiological explanation for learning and how this relates to the other theories of learning. It can be seen that physical well-being, particularly nutrition, is important in enhancing memory and learning and reducing damage.

Section summary

There are numerous pieces of literature which suggest good learning approaches for nurses. There are those that promote adult learning (Sparling 2001), reflection (Cooke & Matarasso 2005), practice (Flanagan et al. 2004), interprofessional team working (Department of Health 1994, 1999; Pollard et al. 2004). All of these learning approaches are based either on a cognitive behavioural approach or a humanistic approach to learning and many employ both views of the nursing student and their learning. These theories of learning are all supported by biological psychologists.

Health promotion

Health promotion is seen as essential within both the UK, from government bodies such as the Department of Health, and the world, with an international impetus from the WHO. Health promotion is considered to be a major element of a nurse's role (NMC 2004), so understanding how people learn or develop their health attitudes, values and behaviours is important for nurses. This understanding can develop from nurses' understanding of how they themselves learn, and applying this to the people with whom they work. This will allow nurses to teach or promote health issues and improve well-being.

> *'Health promotion is the process of enabling people to increase control over, and to improve, their health.' (World Health Organization (WHO), cited Ewles & Simnett 2003, p. 23)*

In the 1980s there was a dispute about the use of the term 'health education' when referring to health promotion, but education still remains a component of the health promotion activity of nurses. The term 'health promotion' is used as it does not have the elements of blame for health problems that occurs with the term 'health education', which could lead to a belief that people become ill because they have not acted on the health education they have received. Health promotion encompasses activities with governments and institutions as well as with the individual.

Whether the term promoting or education is used, much of the activity is to do with learning at an individual, family, organisational and socio-political level. Health promotion should be on the agenda at all levels of society.

Nurses could be involved in the development of understanding and facilitating learning in all areas of society and with all peoples who live within the society whatever their health issues or backgrounds.

Ewles and Simnett (2003, p. 31) offer a framework of health promotion in which nurses may be involved, which includes:

- Health education programmes
- Economic and regulatory activities
- Organisational development
- Community-based work
- Preventive health services (primary, secondary and tertiary)

These require nurses to have good communication skills at all levels and good understanding of not only health-related issues but also how to teach and influence others. As a student nurse there is the need to develop a broad spectrum of basic health promotion skills, but when working as a registered nurse there may be certain areas of health promotion that the nurse focuses on.

Box 3.5   Levels of health promotion

A nurse working with people who have had strokes (cerebro-vascular accidents) may be concerned with promoting health by considering the individual and familial level. They may need to teach the patient and their family about healthy lifestyle activities (preventative health services at a tertiary level) along with rehabilitation techniques to enable speech and mobility (health education programmes). They may need to become involved in dealing with social benefits and access to home aids through government agencies and voluntary agencies. This too may involve educating these agencies about the needs of their client group (organisational development, economic and regulatory activities).

A nurse working with people who have ongoing needs owing to learning disabilities may be promoting health at all levels. They may be involved in teaching clients about healthy eating, exercise, occupation, etc. (preventative health services at primary level) but they may also be dealing with residents, local councils and other government bodies. This might be to ensure that the group of people they are working with has access to appropriate housing and occupation (economic and regulatory activities and community-based work).

The scope of health promotion work for nurses is immense.

Health education programme

Ewles and Simnett (2003) offer some advice to those involved in helping people to learn within health promotion:

- Plan the session beforehand
- Work from the known to the unknown
- Aim for maximum involvement
- Vary learning methods
- Devise learning activities specifically aimed at the group you are helping
- Ensure relevance
- Identify realistic goals
- Use learning contracts
- Evaluate, offer/seek feedback

This can be seen to embrace the cognitive behavioural and humanistic approaches to learning that were identified earlier.

Economic and regulatory activities

Nurses may be involved in lobbying politicians over health-related issues. This is frequently conducted by the nursing professional bodies such as the Royal College of Nurses and the NMC. All nurses, including student nurses, are encouraged to become active in health promotion activities within their unions, to lobby government. If a lobby is to be effective the message needs to be supported by evidence and communicated well. If nurses have a good understanding of communication and learning they should be more effective in this role.

Box 3.6   Example of how nurses might become involved in health promotion at an economic and regulatory level

Nurses may have been involved recently in petitioning government about National Health Service (NHS) reorganisation to food labelling.

Organisational development

Organisations can be of varying size and nurses could be involved in a number, such as a group which supports the clients they work with. Nurses are involved in numerous other organisations such as their unions, the hospital, NHS Trust, prison, school or charity. There are also numerous ways in which nurses become involved in organisational development through health promotion activities.

Box 3.7   Example of how nurses might become involved in health promotion at an organisational level

Many organisations are becoming smoke-free environments due to health promotion messages. Nurses can enhance this development through their health promotion activities, such as teaching coping strategies and offering support for people trying to stop smoking. They can also become involved in policy and procedure developments to ensure optimal health is promoted within the environment, such as infection control techniques and observational policies for clients or patients who are assessed to be at risk.

Community-based work

The health promotion activities that the nurse might become part of in the community should be related to the needs of the community.

Box 3.8   Example of how nurses might become involved in health promotion at a community level

A mental health nurse might recognise that there is limited information and support for people with enduring mental health problems on gaining a fulfilling occupation. They could, with their clients, organise a regular meeting where speakers could be invited to give information and the nurse could enable the clients to support each other.

Preventative health services

This is probably the area where most people would expect nurses to be involved. This area has three sub-sections: primary, secondary and tertiary.

Box 3.9   Primary, secondary and tertiary health promotion

Primary health promotion tends to be focused at people who are not ill; it is focused around services such as well woman clinics, baby clinics, safe sex messages, and child and holiday immunisations.

Secondary health promotion is focused at people who have become unwell and the nurse in this situation would be seeking to assist the person back to a state of health. This can be seen in situations such as the person who has had a myocardial infarction (heart attack), where the nurse seeks to help restore them to health by offering information on healthy living.

Tertiary preventative health promotion would be in situations where a patient or client has ongoing health problems or disability. In the situation where the person has an aggressive cancer, they may be offered palliative care to enhance their quality of life and experience of well-being as a form of health promotion.

All of these areas of health promotion need the nurse to be a good communicator and educator. There is, though, the risk that the nurse is 'forcing' others to accept their understanding of health, which may be at odds with that of other members of the public. Nurses and other health professionals are increasingly being led to offer patient-centred or client-centred care. This can only be done if the nurse has a good understanding of the patient or client's perspective.

It is important that nurses recognise the importance of antidiscriminatory practice and do not assume that the way they perceive the world is the only way to perceive it. The nurse is expected to advocate for those with whom they work (NMC 2004).

Edelman and Mandle (2002) suggest that the nurse's role in health promotion is multifaceted. They suggest the following are the elements of their role:

- Interprofessional team working
- Advocacy
- Care managing
- Consultative
- Delivering services
- Educator
- Healer
- Researcher

Health promoters also use health models to guide their interventions. These are explored in more detail in Chapter 7. It is important to be aware that health psychology research, through the development of health models, has identified elements that might influence behaviour change, which the nurse might be seeking when promoting health. Throughout this section of the chapter both learning and communication have been highlighted as extremely important for nurses in their health promotion role, and one particular health model is useful to nurses in this area.

Ley's model of compliance

Ley (1981, 1989, cited Ogden 2000) developed the cognitive hypothesis model of compliance. This model suggested that there are three elements crucial when considering compliance to treatment: understanding, memory and patient satisfaction. Understanding and memory have an impact on patient satisfaction but all three are directly influential on compliance (see Figure 3.1).

- Understanding – a person needs to understand the treatment and recognise its importance in order to accept the treatment and comply with the regime. This is achieved through learning.
- Memory – if a person cannot remember the dosage or times of treatment etc., they are unlikely to comply with it. Memory and

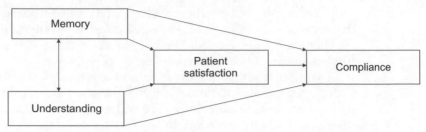

Reproduced from Ogden, *Health Psychology, A Textbook*, © 2004, with kind permission of the Open University Press.

Figure 3.1 Ley's model of compliance.

learning are intrinsically linked, therefore one does not exist without the other.
• Patient satisfaction – patient satisfaction is said to occur when a patient remembers, understands and believes that the person explaining the treatment understands them, their illness and the treatment.

As demonstrated in this model, the learning of the nurse and the patient can be crucial in the patient's acceptance of their care.

Chapter summary

This chapter has demonstrated the need for nurses to be aware of how they learn, so that they can develop their nursing skills and enhance patient or client care. The approaches to learning that each of the psychological perspectives take has been explained and applied to nurses, with the recognition that one of the primary skills that nurses need to learn is people skills.

References

Anderson J.R. (2000) *Cognitive Psychology and its Implications*, 5th edition. New York: Worth Publishers.

Bandura A. (1977) *Social Learning Theory*. Upper Saddle River, NJ: Prentice Hall.

Burnard P. (2002) *Learning Human Skills. An Experiential and Reflective Guide for Nurses and Health Care Professionals*, 4th edition. Oxford: Butterworth Heinemann.

Child D. (1997) *Psychology and the Teacher*, 6th edition. London: Cassell.

Cooke M. & Matarasso B. (2005) Promoting reflection in mental health nursing practice: A case illustration using problem based learning. *International Journal of Mental Health Nursing*, **14**(4), 243–248.

Department of Health (1994) *Working in Partnership: Collaborative Approach to Care*. London: HMSO.

Department of Health (1999) *Making a Difference: Strengthening Nursing, Midwifery and Health Visitor Education*. London: HMSO.

Edelman C.L. & Mandle C.L. (eds) (2002) *Health Promotion Throughout the Lifespan*, 5th edition. London: Mosby.

Ewles L. & Simnett I. (2003) *Promoting Health: a Practical Guide*, 5th edition. London: Bailliere Tindall.

Flanagan B., Nestel D. & Joseph M. (2004) Making patient safety the focus: crisis resource management in the undergraduate curriculum. *Medical Education*, **38**(1), 56–66.

Gagne R.M. (1970) *The Conditions of Learning*, 2nd edition. New York: Holt, Rinehart & Winston.

Johns C. (2000) *Becoming a Reflective Practitioner, a Reflective and Holistic Approach to Clinical Nursing, Practice Development and Clinical Supervision*. Oxford: Blackwell Publishing.

Morrison V. & Bennett P. (2006) *An Introduction to Health Psychology*. London: Pearson, Prentice Hall.

NMC (2004) *Code of Conduct for Nurses*. London: Nursing and Midwifery Council.

Ogden J. (2000) *Health Psychology: A Textbook*, 2nd edition. Buckingham: Open University Press.

Papalia D.E., Feldman R.D. & Olds S.W. (1998) *Human Development*, 7th edition, p. 26. New York: McGraw-Hill.

Pollard K.C., Miers M.E. & Gilchrist M. (2004) Collaborative learning for collaborative working? Initial findings from a longitudinal study of health and social care students. *Health and Social Care in the Community*, **12**(4), 346–358.

Reece I. & Walker S. (1997) *Teaching, Training and Learning: A Practical Guide*, 3rd edition. Sunderland, Tyne and Wear: Business Education Publishers.

Sparling L.A. (2001) Enhancing the learning in self directed learning modules. *Journal for nurses in staff development*, **17**(4), 199–205.

Sweeney N.M., Tucker J., Reynosa B. & Glaser D. (2006) Reducing hunger associated symptoms: the midmorning nutrition break. *Journal of School Nursing*, **22**(1), 32–39.

Understanding Health and Illness through the Lifespan

4

Learning Objectives

An understanding of health and illness throughout the lifespan may appear unnecessary for student nurses within the adult and child branches. This is, though, inaccurate. Every person that is cared for, regardless of age, will not live in a vacuum devoid of contact with other people. They may have grandparents or children whose health and illness will have an impact on them and their well-being. Therefore this chapter is important to all nursing students.

- Discuss a variety of developmental theories and their psychological underpinning.
- Explore how the knowledge of developmental theories can enhance the understanding of the group of people they are caring for.

Identify the underpinning psychological theories for certain nursing interventions.

Introduction

This chapter will focus on how developmental theories such as those of Piaget, Freud, Erikson, and Bowlby inform nursing practice. A case study for each of the branches of nursing – child, adult, mental health and learning disability – will explore the application of some of these theories.

Understanding health and illness

Understandings of health and illness have changed over the years and differ between cultures.

Activity

How would you define health?
How do you think health differs from illness? Is your view the same as the other nurses with whom you work?

Until fairly recently in western societies, a biomedical model of health and illness was held. Within this model, when the body is functioning as it should or as expected, then it is considered to be healthy. When a part of the body is not functioning as it should, the body or person is believed to be ill. If illness were identified within a person, then an appropriate treatment would be found. This treatment should lead to a cure; if it did not the doctor or therapist would consider that they had failed in their role. The biomedical model recognises physical causes for illness. Its approach is to diagnose, provide treatment and seek cure.

This has become problematic within health services as they also include areas such as pregnancy, physical disability, and psychological and behavioural problems. In 1946 the WHO defined health as 'a state of complete physical, mental and social well being not just the absence of disease or infirmity'. This too was problematic in that there was still the assumption that health and illness could be clearly differentiated.

More recently health and illness have been considered to be on a continuum, where the individual's perception of their state of health is important. This led to a new area of psychology developing in the 1980s and 1990s. This new discipline is called health psychology, which seeks to understand health and illness, how people become ill, how they remain well and how they manage chronic ill health and disability.

Health psychologists use a biopsychosocial model to understand health and guide their research. This means they recognise the holistic nature of health; they see health as achieved through an interaction between the biological and psychological functioning within a social arena (see Chapter 7).

Some health issues remain constant throughout the lifespan, such as the need for food, elimination, shelter, oxygen and sleep, but even within these needs there are differences throughout the lifespan. This exploration of health and illness through the lifespan will access various psychological theories, particularly developmental psychological theories. These theories offer nurses the opportunity to understand what might have led to some of those they work with becoming ill, and why others do not.

Developmental theories

Developmental psychology is the field of psychology which focuses on how people change, and ways in which they stay the same over a period of time. It suggests that development is systematic and adaptive and occurs both qualitatively and quantitatively (Papalia et al. 1998).

As identified in Chapter 1, there are five perspectives that guide psychologists in their understanding of the person. Each of these perspectives offers a different understanding of the newborn baby and also how they will develop.

Activity

What do you think a newborn baby's psychological abilities are?
Are they attempting to communicate with others?
Do they have personal desires?
Do they understand the world around them?

Biological psychologists
Biological psychologists believe that biological function and structure determine the individual's behaviour. They suggest that people develop through a sequence of behavioural change determined by maturation of the body, particularly including the nervous and endocrine systems. Individual differences are determined by genes, hormones, neurotransmitters, etc. It is difficult to identify where to start when considering biological developmental theory as the starting point could be the birth of the mother or father, or it could be the release of the egg or fertilisation of the egg or implantation, etc. Given that some psychological theorists do not consider what is happening to the person until birth, that would seem the best starting point. At birth the person is already a complex individual with some sensory and reflexive abilities. Our understanding of biological functioning of the newborn baby is continuing to develop as developing technologies offer more opportunity for insight.

Psychodynamic psychologists

Freud developed this perspective. Psychodynamic psychologists believe that early childhood experience determines future personality. Freud proposed five psychosexual stages. Failure to negotiate a stage results in fixation at that stage. The structure of the mind or psyche is the id, ego and superego. The ego balances the innate impulses of the id and the cultural (learnt) rules of the superego. The personality is influenced by the unconscious mind harbouring repressed memories, which determine conscious thoughts and behaviour (see Chapters 1 and 2).

Behavioural psychologists

Behaviourists believe that learning and experience determine what the person will be like, including their health. They believe that a baby is like a tabula rasa or a blank slate, with only the ability to learn. People learn to be who they are through certain learning processes, such as classical and operant conditioning and social learning. This learning is a continuous process so the behaviourists have little to offer developmental theorists, despite being very useful for understanding health behaviours (see Chapters 1 and 3).

Cognitive psychologists

These psychologists accept that people have learnt to behave in the way they do but are interested in why. They are concerned with thinking or thought processes, to use behavioural terms events that occur between stimulus and response. Some of them have suggested that the human mind is like a computer; it selects, codes, stores and retrieves information. Piaget was a cognitive theorist and he offered a theory of cognitive development, which will be considered later in this chapter.

Humanistic psychologists

The humanists offer a collection of theories about the person but no clear theoretical approach to development over the lifespan. They do, however, accept an inborn motivation to self-actualise, which through learning may be enhanced or interrupted. Despite this, Maslow's hierarchy of needs could be useful throughout the lifespan (see Chapter 1).

Psychodynamic approach to development

Freud proposed five psychosexual stages of development

Freud (founder of the psychodynamic perspective) suggested that development is completed in childhood through five psychosexual stages. Each stage needs to be completed at the appropriate time and if a child was over or understimulated at any stage they might become fixated at that stage and this would dictate their adult personality (see Chapter 2).

The five stages are:

- Oral stage   0–2 years
- Anal stage   2–4 years
- Phallic   4 years to middle childhood
- Latency   middle childhood
- Genital   adolescence through to adulthood

Erikson proposed eight stages of psychosocial development

Erikson was also a psychodynamic theorist and accepted the structure of the mind developed by Freud, but Erikson suggested that development continued throughout life, based on his anthropological studies. He therefore proposed eight stages of development throughout the lifespan. Each stage was labelled a crisis (psychodynamic theories are normative crisis theories – crisis meaning a time of change) which, if successfully resolved, enables the formation of an ego strength or virtue. A successful resolution would be where the positive outcome outweighed the negative outcome but the negative outcome was not completely lost. A complete loss of the negative outcome would also cause problems for the person. He did allow for stages to be revisited, but it would be problematic for the developing person.

Stage 1 – Basic trust versus mistrust
This stage is from birth to 12–18 months old and the baby develops a sense of whether the world is a good and safe place.

It is important to recognise that the theory does not suggest that to have total trust is good; it suggests the need for a balance between trust and mistrust.

Box 4.1   Example of the need for balance between trust and mistrust

If you are caring for an 18-month-old toddler and it trusts everything within the world, it may walk out into the road or reach out to an animal and may suffer serious injury.

If the balance is achieved, the ego strength or virtue of *hope* is gained.

Stage 2 – Autonomy versus shame

In this stage the child is 12–18 months to 3 years old. The child should develop a balance of independence over shame and doubt. In the child's world it is developing internal control, rather than external control previously experienced. Language facilitates the child's striving for autonomy and control as they experience developmental tasks such as toilet training. At this stage also the child is frequently described as going through the 'terrible twos', where the child is attempting to take control but comes into conflict with adult authority.

If the balance is achieved the virtue of *will* is gained.

Stage 3 – Initiative versus guilt

At this stage the child is 3–6 years old. The child develops initiative when trying out new things but should not be overwhelmed by these experiences. The child has divided desires; it desires to achieve new things and be competitive but it also has the desire to be approved of by others, especially its family. The child needs to balance these desires so that it can gain achievements but within the social boundaries.

If the balance is achieved the virtue of *purpose* is gained.

Stage 4 – Industry versus inferiority

The child is now between 6 years old and puberty and must learn skills of the culture or face feelings of incompetence. At this stage the child assesses itself by its productivity and if the child is able to achieve competence in tasks it will develop a high self-esteem.

If achieved, the child will gain the virtue of *skill*.

Stage 5 – Identity versus identity confusion

This stage is called adolescence and the young person is aged from puberty to young adulthood. The adolescent must determine their own sense of self or experience confusion about their roles in life. According to Erikson, this sense of self allows the person to develop intimate relationships in the next stage, to plan for the future and to focus on their goals such as their career, and reduces risk-taking behaviours.

If achieved the young person will gain the virtue or ego strength of *fidelity*.

Stage 6 – Intimacy versus isolation

Young adulthood is where the person seeks to make commitments to others as they develop close intimate relationships to avoid isolation. As people try to develop this relationship they still work to retain their sense of self, developed in the previous stage. If the person successfully achieves this stage they gain a loving relationship while still knowing themselves and having a clear self-concept. If the person is unsuccessful, they may suffer from isolation and self-absorption. Erikson later suggested that women may actually experience stages 5 and 6 the other way round to men. Women were said to find themselves within intimate relationships whereas men need to find themselves first.

If achieved the person will gain the virtue or ego strength of *love*.

Stage 7 – Generativity versus stagnation

Middle adulthood, this crisis is sometimes called the midlife crisis. The mature adult is concerned with establishing and guiding the next generation. There is the need to feel that they are achieving something that is meaningful and that will enhance the well-being of others. If they are unable to do this they can be left with a feeling of personal impoverishment and will become preoccupied with their own needs.

If achieved the person will gain the virtue or ego strength of *care*.

Stage 8 – Integrity versus despair

Late adulthood is where older people need to achieve acceptance of their own life, allowing for the acceptance of death. This acceptance includes acknowledging the things that have not gone well in their lives and their achievements. It is a coming to terms with imperfections of their own humanity and celebrating who they are. If the older person is unable to achieve this, they may experience despair over their inability to relive life and make good their imperfections.

If achieved the person will gain the virtue or strength of *wisdom*.

Attachment theory

What is attachment?

Attachment is an intimate, warm, continuous relationship between mother and baby, where both find satisfaction and enjoyment (Bowlby 1951).

John Bowlby was a child psychiatrist and a psychoanalytic therapist. This means he was medically trained and worked within a psychodynamic perspective. As Bowlby became more interested in attachment, he explored the research of Konrad Lorenz (1966), an ethologist (someone who studies animal behaviour). Lorenz was particularly interested in bonding and imprinting and he identified that for certain animals there was a critical time in which they bonded or imprinted. Ethologists, through their animal studies, originally defined attachment, but Bowlby's work became the defining theory of human attachment. He developed and refined the concept of attachment over a number of years (1958, 1969, 1973, 1980, cited Barnes 1995).

Bowlby, through the work of Lorenz and Freud's psychosexual theory, proposed a critical period for attachment in people of between approximately six months and three years of age. This is when a child needs continuous love and care from one person, the mother or mother substitute. He said that significant separations would have a serious effect on the emotional and social development of the child.

Bowlby said that attachment with the mother is as important for mental health as vitamins and proteins are for physical health (1951). Bowlby proposed that monotropy – the attachment to the mother figure – is qualitatively different from any later attachments. He suggested that without this attachment children would become affectionless psychopaths.

Bowlby (1973) developed a model of how lack of early attachment could have long-term effects on the person. He called this the *internal working model* (see Figure 4.1). He suggested that early life experiences

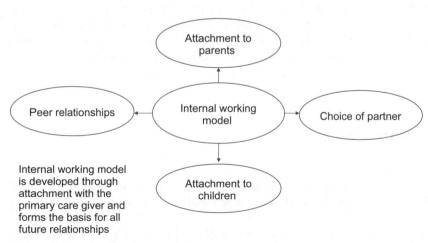

Figure 4.1 Internal working model.

lead the infant to develop beliefs and expectations about the world and relationships. If the infant has received continuous love from its mother it will develop the belief that people can be trusted, that they are worthy of love and that people care. They then carry this forward to future relationships, including their own parenting. These expectations lead to a perception of the world as being benevolent, which is self-reinforcing.

Mary Ainsworth, a student of Bowlby, continued his research on attachment and developed a technique for assessing attachments (the strange situation Ainsworth and Wittig 1969). She found three types of attachment:

- Type A   Anxious – avoidant
- Type B   Securely attached
- Type C   Anxious – resistant

Further research has found that each of these attachment types has implications not only for the child's behaviour but also in predicting adult behaviours.

Bowlby labelled any problems with attachment as deprivation and he did not distinguish between privation and deprivation. Privation is where there has been no opportunity to develop an attachment, such as when a child is in an institution. Deprivation is where the child has developed an attachment but has some separation or loss of that attachment. Privation and deprivation are believed to have different outcomes.

- Deprivation in the short-term could lead to distress but in the long-term to separation anxiety.
- Privation is a long-term problem with the long-term effect of developmental problems or, in Bowlby's term, affectionless psychopathy.

The effects of short-term deprivation are:

- Protest
- Despair
- Detachment

The effects of long-term deprivation – separation anxiety – are:

- Aggressive behaviour
- Clinging behaviour
- Detached behaviour
- Physical health problems

> **Box 4.2   Example of research stimulated by Bowlby's theory**
>
> Bowlby's research influenced the studies of many others, including the Robertsons (1967–73) who through a series of short silent films dramatically changed hospital practice in the care of children. Through these powerful films they demonstrated the impact of depriving a child of its mother over a period of time. This work facilitated the development of parents being allowed to stay in hospital with their children.

The psychodynamically influenced theories of development stress the importance of achieving psychological developmental milestones particularly those in the early years of life.

Cognitive approach to development

Cognitive development is concerned with changes in mental abilities, such as learning, memory, reasoning, thinking and language (Papalia et al. 1998).

Piaget's cognitive theory of development

In the 1930s Piaget suggested that children think in a qualitatively different way from adults, rather than just having less knowledge. He stated that cognitive development occurs through the interaction of innate capabilities with environmental events, and progresses through four distinct hierarchical stages. Piaget's theory is a maturational theory, which utilises the cognitive concept of schemas.

Schema theory

A schema is a building block of intelligent behaviour. Schemas are the mental structures, which provide a mechanism to organise past experiences and to understand new ones (see Chapter 1). Schemas or pockets of knowledge are developed, according to Piaget, through a process of assimilation and accommodation in order to achieve equilibrium.

Assimilation
Assimilation is the incorporation of new information into an existing schema.

Box 4.3 Example of assimilation

You may have a schema of a nurse:

- They work in hospitals
- They care for people who are unwell
- They are kind and helpful
- They are female
- They are young
- They marry doctors

You go into hospital because you are unwell and you are introduced to your nurse and he is male. You now need to adjust your schema because nurses are also male – this is assimilation. When assimilation has occurred you are psychologically restored to equilibrium.

Accommodation
Accommodation is where an existing schema needs to be changed or a new one developed to include new information.

Box 4.4 Example of accommodation

We will return to your schema of a nurse:

- They work in hospitals
- They care for people who are unwell
- They are kind and helpful
- They are female or male
- They are young
- They marry doctors

You start your nursing course and find that nurses do not all work in hospitals, only a few nurses marry doctors, and nurses are aged from 18 to 65. At this point disequilibrium occurs and to regain equilibrium the schema needs to be changed or adapted – this is called accommodation.

Piaget's four stages of cognitive development

- Sensori-motor stage   0–2 years old
- Pre-operational stage   2–7 years old

- Concrete operations   7–11 years old
- Formal operations   11 years onwards

Sensori-motor stage

At this first stage of development, physical schemas are being created and there are six sub-stages.

Sub-stage 1
The baby is from birth to 1 month and the stage is labelled *reflexive activity* as the activities or physical schemas used are reflexive. Infants are refining their innate responses, for example, sucking.

Sub-stage 2
The baby now is 1–4 months old and this stage is labelled primary circular reactions. This is where actions which happened by chance are repeated when something has been gained, for example moving thumb to mouth to suck it. The baby has no sense of object permanence, which means that if something does not stimulate the senses of the baby it does not exist.

Sub-stage 3
The infant is now 4–8 months old and this stage is labelled secondary circular reactions. The infant is using established schemata (plural of schema) to explore new objects, for example the baby will suck a new toy it is given.

Sub-stage 4
The infant is now 8–12 months old and the stage is labelled co-ordination of secondary schemata. The young child is co-ordinating previously learned schemas and is able to use learned behaviour to achieve goals, for example the baby will push things out of the way to get to a toy. At this stage they have some sense of object permanence, hence the seeking out of toys.

Sub-stage 5
At 12–18 months old the toddler is in the stage labelled tertiary circular reactions. At this time the young child uses trial and error strategies to obtain goals, and babies experiment with objects, for example dropping them out of their pushchair and then looking for them.

Sub-stage 6
The 18–24 month-old-child is expected to now be in the stage labelled 'new means through mental combinations'. Symbolic activity starts to appear: a child can use a sound or action to represent an object not there, for example making the noise and action of an aeroplane. They show signs of problem solving and have a sense of object permanence (Davey 2004).

Pre-operational stage

At the pre-operational stage the child at the age of 2–7 years has made some qualitatively different thinking achievements:

- Uses representational systems, for example words
- Understanding of cause and effect (understanding why things happen)
- Ability to classify
- Understanding of number concepts
  - 1 to 1 principle (each item has one number)
  - stable-order principle (numbers always go in set order – 1,2,3,4 . . .)
  - order-irrelevance principle (it does not matter where you start, you still have the same number of the given items)
  - cardinality principle (the last number said when counting the number of items)
  - abstraction principle (counting can be applied to many things).

Limitations
There continue to be a number of limitations to the thinking abilities of the child at this stage (Papalia et al. 1998, p. 196):

- Centration – inability to decentre, the child can only focus on one element at a time
- Conservation – number, length, liquid, matter, weight, area; the child does not recognise that number etc. will stay the same if the local environment changes
- Inability to distinguish appearance from reality
- Irreversibility – fails to see an action can go both ways
- Transductive reasoning – sees cause where none exists
- Egocentrisim – assumes everyone thinks as they do
- Animism – attributes life to inanimate objects

> **Case study Demonstrating pre-operational thought**
>
> A child of five is watching you care for their mother and asks you how long you are going to be visiting them. You explain that you will be visiting for the next five days and show them the days on the calendar. The child happily counts the days (demonstrating stable-order principle), starting at the first day you showed them and then they start with the last day, and are happy they have understood you are coming for five days (demonstrating order-irrelevance principle). They go on to ask you whether your mother will be upset at you visiting them for five days (demonstrating egocentrism and centration). You explain that you will come to visit them for an hour each day and then go home afterwards. The child then says, but how can you go home and come back (irreversibility). You explain that you will go home in your car, and show them your car outside. The child then brightly exclaims, as if finally under-standing, that you cannot stay with them because your car would be sad (animism and transducive reasoning), but that you will come back in five days.

Concrete operations

When a child reaches the concrete operational stage at 7–11 years old they are able to achieve thinking that had not been available to them in the pre-operational stage. They have the ability to (Papalia et al. 1998):

- Conserve.
- Classify – class inclusion (an object can be in more than class).
- Serialise – organisation of darkest to lightest.
- Do more complex thinking but still remaining within the concrete world number and mathematics – for example Jenny went to the shop with 15 pence and spent 10 pence on sweets. How much did she have left?
- Distinguish between fantasy and reality.

Formal operations

From the age of 11 onwards, children develop adult thinking processes allowing greater imagination and abstract thinking. They have the ability to use hypothetical deductive reasoning and can manipulate ideas or propositions.

Application of developmental theory to nursing branches

Children's nursing scenario

Case study   Jade

You are working on the children's ward of your local hospital. Jade, aged two, has had to come into hospital for an operation and her mother has been unable to stay with her as she has two other children, one older and one younger than Jade. Jade's mother had stayed while Jade had the operation and was there when she woke up, but had to leave afterwards to see to the other children. During this first day Jade was happy to have you play with her on her bed, check her wound, temperature, pulse, etc. The following day you hear from the night staff that Jade spent most of the night in tears asking for her mother, and this morning she is refusing to allow anyone to offer her food or comfort and appears hot and bothered. Some members of the team suggest she is behaving badly and is spoilt, while other members of the team express their concern. As you had previously had a good relationship with her, the senior nurse asks you to develop Jade's care plan and present this to the nursing team, explaining your reasons.

Initial assessment shows that Jade is refusing food and touch and appears hot and distressed. Jade at the moment will not allow you to undertake any further investigations.

Activity

What theories might help you understand Jade's behaviour?
How would these theories guide your interventions with Jade?

At two years old Jade is still within the critical time period, described by Bowlby, when the child needs a continuous relationship with her mother to maintain a secure attachment. This will help Jade develop an internal working model that people can have warm, secure and trusting relationships. She should have developed an attachment for her mother at two and may be experiencing short-term deprivation. This has three stages: protest, despair and detachment. It can clearly be seen in Jade's behaviour that she is in stage one – protest. This offers an explanation for Jade's behaviour, but how will it inform your interventions?

Some suggested interventions:

- Ask the mother to bring in things that are familiar for Jade – toys, clothes, etc.
- Have a photograph of Jade's mother for her to look at.
- Encourage visiting by other people that Jade knows well.
- Keep routines that Jade had at home.
- Talk to Jade about her mother.

Another psychodynamic theorist that may enhance understanding of Jade's behaviour is Erkison. He suggested that at two years old Jade would be in stage two of his psychosocial developmental theory. At this stage children are developing autonomy over shame and doubt. If they progress successfully they will gain will. This is a time when children are attempting to become independent and take control over their bodies and their worlds. It is known as a time called the 'terrible twos' and can be a time when mothers struggle with their children's temper when they do not get what they want. Jade may be feeling unable to control her body and environment; this could release disruptive behaviour.

Some suggested interventions:

- Make boundaries clear so that Jade can take control within safe limits.
- Discuss and explain decisions to Jade.
- Ask Jade for her permission to do activities or interventions.
- When Jade loses control of herself ensure the environment is safe.
- Give space to Jade to regain her dignity after she has lost control.
- Offer activities that can occupy Jade, distract her and allow her to makes successes.

At the age of two Jade would fall into the pre-operational stage of cognitive development founded by Piaget. Piaget suggested that children think in a qualitatively different way from adults; it is not just that they have fewer thoughts. According to this theory Jade would not be able to understand a different point of view from her own; she would be egocentric. She would be able to focus on only one element at a time (centration) and may see causes where none exist (transductive reasoning), for example she may believe that her mother has left her in hospital because she does not want her. Along with transductive reasoning, she may be unable to see that things can be reversed or to distinguish appearance from reality. As her mother is not there she may be unable to believe her mother will return. If Jade is unable to understand why her mother has left her (ego centrism) and unable to understand that she will return (irreversibility) and thinks that it is her fault (ego centrism), her distress can easily be understood.

Some suggested interventions:

* Offer reasons for her mother's departure and return.
* Speak to Jade in a language she can understand.
* Use diagrams and calendars etc. to explain and gain understanding from Jade.

Behavioural and biological theories may also offer an understanding of Jade's behaviour. Social learning theory may offer an explanation of Jade's behaviour in terms of learning. It might suggest that Jade has learnt by observing and imitating others' distress behaviour to gain comfort. She may feel discomfort due to emotional or physical reasons and has learnt that to behave distressed will engage others into providing for her needs.

Some suggested interventions:

* Offer Jade and the other children comfort, whether they appear to need it or not.
* Reassure Jade that you want to help her.

Biologically Jade may be in physical or emotional pain due to her operation and may feel nauseous due to this, which would encourage her to refuse food. When in pain she may feel afraid of being touched as this may increase the pain. This may be due to the healing process, but may be due to healing not progressing well.

Some suggested interventions:

* Offer Jade reassurance that you want to help her feel better.
* Show her what you want to do prior to doing it.
* Investigate physical health state: check for pain, temperature, and nausea.
* Move slowly and allow her to do what she can of the physical checks.

Summary

Psychological theory can offer insights into the behaviour of children when they are ill and when they are well. This scenario has considered the psychodynamic theories of Bowlby and Erikson, along with the cognitive theory of Piaget and the biological and behavioural theories, in an attempt to understand Jade's behaviour. The interventions suggested for each of the approaches are not exclusive and in fact most psychologists and nurses work in an eclectic manner, developing interventions for individual people from more than one theoretical approach.

Adult nursing scenario

Case study   John

You are caring for John, a man of 50, who has recently had a myo-cardial infarction (MI). In the first hours after his heart attack he appeared to have been pleased he had survived and full of enthu-siasm to start his rehabilitation. Two days later he asks for food to be brought to him in bed, he refuses to have a shower or to move from his bed and is constantly pressing the nurse call button com-plaining of chest pain. When encouraged to do anything for himself he becomes verbally aggressive.

Activity

How might other members of staff view John's behaviour? Would he be seen as a difficult patient?

According to Erikson's psychosocial theory, John would be in middle adulthood – a period of generativity versus stagnation. At this stage people are striving to develop and guide the next generation and if they are successful they achieve the ego strength or virtue of care. For John at the moment this may feel as if it has been taken away from him and he may no longer feel he can play a useful role in the development of others. Also at this stage, men frequently reappraise their lives and look for new opportunities, which he may now believe are unavailable to him. As his physical state has deteriorated, his self-esteem may have fallen. Given this approach to viewing John's situation, he may be seen as withdrawing and stagnating to protect himself, and using aggres-sion as a maladaptive coping strategy when encouraged to participate in his rehabilitation.

Some suggested interventions:

- Discuss with John what his hopes for the future are.
- Offer health information about what he may be able to undertake in the future given his health problems.
- Identify with John what developmental activities with his chil-dren/colleagues etc. he had been undertaking prior to his health problem and reassure him about what he may be able to achieve in the future.
- Ask John to talk to other people about something he has experi-enced, to support them.

Another psychdynamic theory that may offer some understanding for John's behaviour is Bowlby's attachment theory. Bowlby suggests that people, when they are small children, develop an internal working model of the world including other people. John may have developed an internal working model that people cannot be trusted and the world is an unsafe place. This may have developed through an insecure attachment to his mother in the first two years of his life. This might lead John not to trust the nursing staff when they reassure him about his safety and ability to undertake self-care tasks such as showering. Insecure attachment may also lead John not to trust himself and his abilities, as he has not developed the self-reassuring as a small child.

Some suggested interventions:

- Give John opportunities to trust himself
  - Set small achievable goals so that John can recognise his successes
  - Highlight John's achievements to him
- Demonstrate your trustworthiness
  - Ensure you do not make promises you cannot keep – if you say you will get something for him now, do so
  - Do not make statements that cannot be evidenced.

Social learning theory could also offer insights into John's behaviour. This would suggest that he has learnt the behaviour by watching and imitating other people. John could have learnt in childhood that if people do not behave as if they are ill (the above could be seen as illness behaviour), then they will not receive the care they need. Or he may have seen another person who enthusiastically engaged in rehabilitation early in the recover stage and then became very poorly, either while he has been in hospital or before his health problem. This may lead John to protect himself from nursing staff who try to encourage him to self-care and mobilise.

Some suggested interventions:

- Give John time to express his concerns.
- Give John the opportunity to speak to others who have had similar problems and are progressing well.
- Allow John to observe others progressing through their rehabilitation.
- Reassure John about his recovery.

There may also be a biomedical explanation for John's behaviour. It may be that he is experiencing undisclosed pain. He may be having angina post-MI that is making it painful for him to move. Owing to pain John could behave quite irritably due to the discomfort and fear (see Chapter 7).

Some suggested interventions:

- Ask John if he is in pain.
- John may be predisposed to heart problems or hypersensitive to pain, so check family history.
- If you are concerned that he is in pain, refer him to the doctor or nurse prescriber.
- Offer non-medication pain relief approaches, such as relaxation and aromatherapy.
- Discuss your concerns with the interprofessional team (doctor, occupational therapist, physiotherapist, etc.).

Summary

A number of psychological theories could explain John's present behaviour and the interventions that each would lead to. These are not mutually exclusive. Nurses and psychologists in clinical practice tend to work in an eclectic manner dependent on the needs of the individual.

Learning disability nursing scenario

Case study   Martha

You are working with a woman named Martha who is 30 years old. She grew up in local authority accommodation and when she left compulsory schooling she was given some support for independent living by a social worker. Martha has few friends but is known in the local community as she frequently smells of body odour or strong perfume and is seen as clumsy. Despite her difficulties Martha had been working part-time in a local charity shop, which she enjoyed, but it had to close. She has recently come to the attention of the learning disability nursing team. This was due to the police being called to her flat on a number of occasions, as she was very frightened by her neighbours who had been shouting at her.

Martha was a poorly child and frequently in and out of hospital. She has been diagnosed with epilepsy, an IQ of 60 and poor visio-spatial ability (she sometimes bumps into things). Martha attended a mainstream school but was isolated and did not undertake any qualifications. Martha's mother was a single teenager when she gave birth to Martha, but despite her attempts she could not cope with caring for a child as well as herself. Martha was initially taken into foster care but after a few unsuccessful placements she eventually settled in the local authority accommodation.

> **Activity**
>
> Do you think that Martha's learning disability is the cause of her problems?
>
> Do you think there may be some other reason for Martha's present difficulties?

Bowlby's attachment theory may offer some understanding of Martha's present problems. He suggests that people need a warm, loving, continuous relationship with their mother or mother substitute for the first 3 years of their life. This was obviously not the situation for Martha; her mother struggled initially and then Martha moved from home to home, which would not facilitate the development of a continuous, warm, loving relationship. Martha's internal working model would be a world where people could not be trusted and her sense of being a valuable person would not have been developed. Bowlby says that without this attachment people will struggle with their mental health and social skills. This can be seen to be the case for Martha; her social skills are lacking and her mental health is at risk (she is fearful and has problems learning).

Some suggested interventions:

- Develop an ongoing trusting relationship with Martha.
- Take time to find out what Martha would like to achieve, treating her with respect.
- Explore how Martha can continue to live in her accommodation without fear.

Another psychodynamic theory of development that may help understand Martha's situation is Erikson's psychosocial theory. Erikson outlined an eight-stage theory of development across the whole lifespan. Martha can be seen to have had difficulties with each stage she should have experienced.

Stage 1 – Trust versus mistrust
As Martha was moved from one care giver to another she would have had difficulty developing hope, which is the ego strength or virtue at this stage.

Stage 2 – Autonomy versus shame
It is difficult to assess Martha's opportunity to develop will, but Erikson says that although a person can move on to another stage without achieving the one before, it will be more problematic for them.

Stages 3 and 4 – Initiative versus guilt and industry versus inferiority
These may both have been a problem for Martha due to her learning disability and her ongoing health problems. This may have resulted in her struggling to achieve purpose and skill.

Stages 5 and 6 – Identity versus identity confusion and intimacy versus isolation
These may also have been problematic for Martha as she had limited opportunity to develop a sense of self at school and she has few friends. This may lead Martha to have limited fidelity and love.

All of these issues may have led to the need for the learning disability nurses to become involved in supporting her back to independent living.
Some suggested interventions:

- Develop an ongoing trusting relationship with Martha.
- Identify what Martha enjoys and her skills.
- Access adult education.
- Support Martha seeking new employment.

Behaviourism and social learning theory could also help understand Martha's situation. The behaviourists believe that every thing a person does and is perceived to be is due to learning. Therefore, if there are any problems with Martha's behaviour it is due to faulty learning. Some of this learning is more voluntary, as in operant conditioning where people are rewarded for certain behaviours, which then encourages them to repeat the behaviour. Other behaviours are less voluntary and are learnt through classical conditioning; these are more reflex-like behaviours. Social learning theory takes this learning approach to another level by proposing that people learn by observation and imitation (vicarious learning). Therefore Martha may have learnt to deal with body odour by increasing the amount of perfume she wears. Also, vicarious learning and operant conditioning may have taught Martha to be fearful of her neighbours and she may not have learnt how to regain employment.
Some suggested interventions:

- Become a role model for Martha.
- Support Martha's learning in areas such as personal hygiene, social skills and employment skills.
- Facilitate the development of adaptive coping strategies.

Piaget's cognitive theory of development can also offer some understanding of Martha's situation. This theory is maturational and depends on innate capabilities and experience from the environment. At each stage the child's thoughts are qualitatively different. Given Martha's situation, she may be thought to have innate limitations given her IQ (although this is debatable) and limited environmental opportunities. This may lead to Martha being stuck at a lower maturational cognitive level. She may not be able to proceed to formal operations and may only be able to think at a more concrete operational level or even pre-operational. If this is so Martha could have problems with centration (focusing on one thing at a time), which may include understanding other people's points of view or manipulating thoughts in her head. If these are a problem for Martha she may have problems interpreting her neighbours and the impact she has on others by her personal hygiene strategies.

Some suggestions for interventions:

- Focus on one problem at a time with Martha, taking small steps to achieve larger goals.
- Increase Martha's social environment to allow her to develop her cognitive abilities.
- Facilitate Martha's opportunities for experiencing other physical and mental challenges.

A biological explanation could also be offered to understand Martha's situation. Given her mother's age and ability to cope, Martha may have been undernourished both inter-uterine and post-birth. This may have a significant impact on her ability to learn, along with having ongoing health problems such as epilepsy, which had led to frequent hospitalisation. Her learning problems may also be due to a genetic problem. It has also been found that lack of stimulation in early life reduces the opportunity for nervous system and brain growth, which could also lead to problems with learning as the child grew, and into adulthood.

Some suggestions for interventions:

- Ensure optimal physical environment for learning, such as warmth, balanced diet, sleep and safety.
- Ensure epilepsy is optimally managed.
- Provide learning opportunities for Martha when she has the greatest sense of well-being.

Summary

A number of psychological theories could explain Martha's present situation, and the interventions that each would lead to are not mutually exclusive. Nurses and psychologists in their caring environment tend to work in an eclectic manner dependent on the needs of the individual.

Mental health nursing scenario

Case study Mary

You are working with a woman named Mary who is 30 years old. She has been receiving intermittent care from mental health services since she was 17 years old, when she had taken an overdose of paracetamol. Mary disclosed to the mental health nurse that her stepfather, in whose care she had been since she was three years old when her mother left them, had been sexually abusing her. Mary has received a number of diagnoses over the years but presently has the diagnosis of borderline personality disorder. She has problems making and keeping relationships and those caring for her find her difficult to engage in a therapeutic manner and they believe her to be manipulative. She frequently feels low in mood, occasionally hears voices and when she becomes distressed she uses self-harm as a coping strategy. When Mary finds life too difficult she self-harms by cutting her abdomen, but if this is not effective in reducing her distress she takes overdoses of her prescribed medication.

Bowlby's attachment theory could offer some insight into Mary's situation. He suggests that people need a warm, loving, continuous relationship with their mother or mother substitute for the first three years of their life. This may not have been the situation for Mary as her mother left her at this time. Mary may have developed an internal working model of a world where people could not be trusted, and her sense of being a valuable person would not have been developed. This would have been compounded by the abuse of her stepfather after this time. This internal working model could lead Mary to have problems with adult relationships and to have feelings of low self-worth, perhaps self-hatred. Mary's self-harm could be understood in this context. Bowlby says that without this attachment people will become affectionless psychopaths.

Some suggested interventions:

- Develop an ongoing trusting relationship with Mary.
- Give Mary opportunities to trust herself:
  - Set small achievable goals so that Mary can recognise her successes.
  - Highlight Mary's achievements to her.

- Demonstrate your trustworthiness:
  - Ensure that you do not make promises you cannot keep – if you say you will get something for her now, do so.
  - Do not make statements that cannot be evidenced.
- Take time to find out what Mary hopes to achieve, treating her with respect.

Another psychodynamic theory of development that may help understand Mary's situation is Erikson's psychosocial theory. Erikson outlined an eight-stage theory of development across the whole lifespan. Mary could have had difficulties with each stage she should have experienced.

Stage 1 – Trust versus mistrust
Mary's relationship with her mother may have been problematic and she was abandoned, so she may have had difficulty developing hope, which is the ego strength or virtue at this stage.

Stage 2 – Autonomy versus shame
It is difficult to assess Mary's opportunity to develop will, but as her mother left without Mary having any control and she was being abused, she may have developed a sense of shame rather than will.

Stage 3 – Initiative versus guilt
This may have been a problem as this is a time of developing competitiveness within social boundaries. As Mary was abused, which is a breach of social boundaries, she may have developed guilt instead of purpose.

Stage 4 – Industry versus inferiority
It is difficult to know if this was a problem for Mary but Erikson says that if a person has had problems achieving the earlier ego strengths, then the next will be harder to achieve. Therefore Mary may be struggling with her self-esteem.

Stages 5 and 6 – Identity versus identity confusion and intimacy versus isolation
These may also have been problematic for Mary as she had limited opportunity to develop a sense of self and intimacy due to the abusive relationship. This may lead Mary to have limited fidelity and love and may create her current relationship problems.

Some suggested interventions:

- Develop an ongoing trusting relationship with Mary.
- Demonstrate your trustworthiness:
  - Ensure you do not make promises you cannot keep – if you say you will get something for her now, do so.
  - Do not make statements that cannot be evidenced.
- Take time to find out what Mary hopes to achieve, treating her with respect.
- Identify what Mary enjoys and her skills.
- Set small achievable goals so that Mary can recognise her successes.
- Highlight Mary's achievements to her.
- Offer Mary group therapy to develop her social relationship skills.
- If Mary is in a relationship at present, offer relationship counselling.

Behaviourism and social learning theory could also help understand Mary's situation. The behaviourists believe that everything a person does and is perceived to be, is due to learning. Therefore if there are any problems with Mary's behaviour it is due to faulty learning. Some of this learning is more voluntary, as in operant conditioning where people are rewarded for certain behaviours, which then encourages them to repeat the behaviour. Other behaviours are less voluntary and are learnt through classical conditioning; these are more reflex-like behaviours. Social learning theory takes this learning approach to another level in proposing that people learn by observation and imitation (vicarious learning). Therefore Mary may have learnt that if she harms herself she will get the care she feels she needs. She may also have learnt that affection is only achieved through sexual relationships, and is therefore unsure of social boundaries and her relationships fail.

Some suggested interventions:

- Become a role model for Mary.
- Support Mary's learning.
- Facilitate the development of adaptive coping strategies.

A biological explanation could also be offered to understand Mary's situation. Mary may have a genetic predisposition to mental health problems or her mother may have become ill during pregnancy. She may also have had some neuro-chemical changes, which have interfered with her ability to perceive situations accurately.

Some suggestions for interventions:

- Ensure an optimal physical environment for Mary such as warmth, balanced diet, sleep and safety.
- Refer Mary to have an assessment for medication.
- Refer Mary for scans to check for structural brain changes.

Summary

A number of psychological theories could explain Mary's present situation, and the interventions that each would lead to are not mutually exclusive. Nurses and psychologists in their caring environment tend to work in an eclectic manner dependent on the needs of the individual.

Chapter summary

This chapter has considered the major developmental theories in psychology and has offered some indication on how these can influence health. The second part of the chapter has discussed a case study for each of the nursing branches, to identify how they can support nursing understanding and guide interventions.

References

Ainsworth M. & Wittig B.A. (1969) Attachment and exploratory behaviour of one-year-olds in a strange situation. In: Foss B.M. (ed.) *Determinants of Infant Behaviour*, vol. 4. London: Methuen.

Barnes, P. (ed) (1995) *Personal, Social and Emotional Development of Children*, p. 5. Oxford: Blackwell Publishers.

Bowlby J. (1951) Maternal care and mental health. *Bulletin of the World Health Organization*, 3, 355–535.

Bowlby J. (1973) *Separation. Attachment and Loss*, vol 2. Harmondsworth: Penguin.

Davey G. (2004) *Complete Psychology*, p. 301. Oxford: Hodder & Stoughton.

Lorenz K. (1996) *On Aggression*. London: Methuen.

Papalia D.E., Feldman R.D. & Olds S.W. (1998) *Human Development*, 7th edition. New York: McGraw-Hill.

Robertson J. & Robertson J. (1967–73) *Young Children in Brief Separation*. Film series, no 3 (1969): John 17 months, 9 days in a residential nursery. London: Tavistock.

World Health Organization (1946) *World Health Organization Constitution*. Geneva: WHO.

Psychological Theory for Nursing in a Social World

Learning Objectives

All nursing occurs in a social world; nursing care may be offered in a wide variety of environments but all are essentially social. It is therefore important that nurses are aware not only of their own actions but also of how they understand and interact with others.

- Using psychological theories, explain how nurses may understand other people's behaviour.
- Discuss how nurses and patients may develop their attitudes, and why and how these might be changed.
- Identify how nurses might understand their relationships and why an understanding of self-concept is an important element of this.

Introduction

This chapter initially focuses on how nurses form an understanding of their own and other people's behaviour through what is known as attribution theories. These theories offer explanations of how a nurse may make judgements and predictions about the behaviour of those with whom they work. The next section explores attitudes, how these develop, their function and how and why nurses may seek to change them. Once the psychological theories that enhance the understanding of working with individuals have been considered, the chapter moves on to use psychological theory to understand how people work together as groups. Finally, the chapter finishes by returning to understanding oneself in a social context and individual relationships.

Attribution theories

Attribution theories offer psychologists and nurses an understanding of how people interpret other people's behaviour. This is important, as it will help nurses understand the common mistakes that they might make and that others might make as naïve psychologists.

Fritz Heider (1958, cited Hogg & Vaughan 1998) suggested that people seek to understand others' behaviour and, given the techniques they use for doing this, are similar to social psychologists; he labelled them 'naive scientists'. He based this view on three main points:

- People believe that their behaviour is motivated and therefore seek motivations in others' behaviour.
- People tend to seek to understand the causes of events within the world and so seek stable features, in order to identify causal relationships, and they also do this with others.
- People, when seeking causal relationships, try to identify whether an event is environmental (external) or person-related (internal).

These premises became the foundation of future attribution theories, such as Jones and Davis's theory of correspondent inference, Kelley's covariation model and Weiner's attributional theory.

Jones and Davis's theory of correspondent inference

A correspondent inference is where a decision is made as to whether a person's behaviour appears to be related to an underlying predisposition; the behaviour corresponds or is attributed to a personality trait.

Jones and Davis suggest people use clues to determine whether the behaviour is related to the underlying personality. The clues are:

- Choice – was the person able to choose to behave in this manner?
- Social desirability – was the behaviour predictable due to social norms or expectations?
- Roles – was the person just doing what was expected of them given their role?
- Prior expectation – was the behaviour typical of the person?

If the behaviour was typical of the person and not merely due to social convention or their role, and they had a choice in performing the behaviour, it would be attributed to their internal disposition or personality (Gross 2001).

Box 5.1   Example of correspondent interference

As a nurse is going home after working her shift, and is sat in the waiting area awaiting a colleague to whom she is giving a lift home, she hears one patient telling another that they have bought their granddaughter a birthday card, but as the birthday is tomorrow it will not get there in time. They go on to say it is a pity as their granddaughter only lives a few streets away. The colleague arrives to see that the nurse is explaining that she would be happy to deliver the card on her way home. The nurse had the *choice* to offer to help; it was not part of her *role* and although it was *socially desirable*, it was not *expected*. Given that the nurse had already offered them a lift home, the colleague believed this was *typical* of the nurse and therefore attributed the nurse to having a kind and generous disposition.

Kelley's covariance model (1967, cited Carlson et al. 2004)

This theory of attribution is similar to Jones and Davis's theory of attribution in that it suggests that people seek to establish whether a behaviour is due to an internal cause or a situational one. Unlike the clues that are used with Jones and Davis's theory, Kelley's model says that people attribute behaviour using three aspects:

- Consensus – do other people react in the same way as this person?
- Consistency – is this a response the person usually makes in this situation?
- Distinctiveness – does this behaviour occur frequently or is it distinct to this situation?

If a behaviour is consistently (consistency) enacted by this person and occurs across situations (it lacks distinctiveness) and is not something that most other people would do in this situation (lacks consensus), the behaviour is attributed to an internal dispositional cause.

> **Box 5.2 Example of covariance attribution**
>
> Each time (*consistency*) Tom, a mental health nurse, has to administer an injection to his clients, he takes with him an information leaflet, which he explains and offers to the client before giving the injection. This is to ensure they understand what is being given to them and that he has gained informed consent. The other nurses he works with verbally explain, and offer the leaflet if requested (lack of *consensus*). Tom always uses the same approach regardless of the medication that is being administered, and he does the same thing with any other interventions he carries out (lacking in *distinctiveness*). This behaviour then would be considered to be due to his internal disposition.

Although Heider suggested that people were naive scientists, they tend to be less logical than the attributional theories above would suggest and biases in attribution can be seen. These occur through personality or interpersonal dynamics, or can be biased to meet individual needs (Hogg & Vaughan 1998).

This has led to the development of the fundamental attribution error identified by Ross (1977, cited Hogg & Vaughan 1998). This suggests that people are usually biased towards attributing others' behaviour to internal depositions, whereas they tend to attribute their own behaviours to external factors. There are a number of hypotheses about explaining this tendency:

- Focus of attention – people tend to watch people not the environment.
- Differential forgetting – people forget the environmental factors more quickly than other people's behaviour.
- Cultural and developmental factors – young children do not make this sort of error but develop the attribution of dispositional factors as they grow and learn the cultural norms, and it is not consistent across cultures.
- Linguistic factors – the English language facilitates describing dispositions of the person, not the environment

The tendency to attribute others' behaviour to internal factors and our own to external factors has been labelled the actor – observer effect. This has been said to occur due to either perceptual focus or informational differences.

Box 5.3 Example of the actor–observer effect

I observe one of my nursing colleagues being thanked and praised by a patient's relative. I wonder what they have done that has pleased the relative; perhaps they were kind towards a patient (attributing behaviour to internal disposition).

The next day I am approached by the same relative who shakes my hand and thanks me for the care that has been given to their relative, saying that they are looking so much better day on day. I have not provided any care for their relative. I gracefully accept the thanks on behalf of the nursing team but recognise that the praise was not due to my efforts but care that others had provided (attributing behaviour to external factors). This actor–observer effect can be seen to be due to my having more information about my behaviour, and also my initial attribution could be due to my focus on the other nurse rather than on the situation – they did not enter or leave the area where the relative came from.

Section summary

This part of the chapter has considered how nurses might make causal attributions – how they decide what has caused a person to behave in the way they have. This could in turn affect how attractive the person is seen to be, whether they are a nurse or a person needing nursing care, which will influence how that care is accepted or provided. It has also considered people to be naïve scientists, and also factors that might influence inaccuracies within their decision-making.

Attitudes

Allport (1935) described attitude as the single most indispensable concept in social psychology, and its relevance in the study of health and healthcare cannot be overestimated. Despite this, the study of attitudes is fraught with problems. This will be explored within this section of this chapter.

Definitions

Attitude:

> *'a mental or neural state of readiness, organised through experience, exerting a directive or dynamic influence upon the individual's response to all objects and situations with which it is related.' (Allport 1935)*

Beliefs:

'what we hold to be true about the world, which often form a coherent or complex value system, for example religious or political beliefs. Beliefs are more deeply held than attitudes, and represent what we think of as true about the world.' (Pennington et al. 1999, p. 72)

Values:

'. . . represent our ethical and moral codes of conduct, highly influenced by our cultural, social and peer group norms. Again, often deeply held and resistant to change, and may affect attitudes, values are usually strongly related to beliefs.' (Pennington et al. 1999, p. 72)

Box 5.4   Examples of values, beliefs and attitudes

While a nurse is caring for the mother of a 14-year-old girl, the mother tells the nurse that her daughter is pregnant and that she is trying to persuade her daughter to have the pregnancy terminated. The nurse listens and demonstrates care and concern for the woman, and offers some suggestions as how she could support her daughter in making the decision. The nurse demonstrated a caring *attitude* towards the woman despite the nurse's *belief* that terminating a pregnancy was unacceptable. Despite personal beliefs, the nurse's attitude was influenced by the *values* developed through professional respect for the biomedical ethical principles.

There is an interrelationship between attitudes, values and beliefs and all are very difficult to alter. Attitudes could be considered the emotional, cognitive and behavioural response to beliefs influenced by the values of the person. Despite this, attitudes have been found to be the most easily of the three to be changed, as we will find later in the chapter.

Functions of attitude

Katz (1960, cited Gross 2001) offers four major functions of attitudes:

- Knowledge function – Attitudes offer a framework for experience and a type of short-cut, reducing the mental effort involved in assessing a situation or response.
- Adjustive function – This is where a person may exhibit an attitude that does not relate to their beliefs but is socially acceptable, as could be said of the example above.

- Value-expressive function – This occurs when a person expresses an attitude that correlates strongly with an important value and allows the person to demonstrate personal integrity.
- Ego-defensive function – Attitudes can help protect people by allowing them to deny or avoid self-knowledge.

Pratkanis and Greenwald (1989, cited Hogg & Vaughan 1998) suggest that attitudes have three functions. They:

- Allow the person to make sense of the world
- Offer an heuristic or simple strategy for understanding an object
- Provide a schema to organise and guide the memory

According to Hogg and Vaughan (1998) and Pennington et al. (1999), attitudes influence people's thoughts, feelings and behaviours in many areas, such as lifestyle choices, consumer activity, voting and political behaviour, even interpersonal attraction.

In healthcare and nursing, the impact of attitudes on those providing care and those receiving care is significant and could possibly precipitate:

- Fear of hospitals, doctors, nurses or various medical treatments
- Awe of doctors and nurses, which may lead to submissive behaviour and lack of autonomy
- A negative response to health information, such as smoking cessation and safe sex
- Prejudice towards certain groups of people, such as people who self-harm, are obese or have a learning disability

Attitude formation

There are a number of theories of attitude development from behavioural theories, including classical conditioning, operant conditioning, social learning theory (see Chapters 1 and 3) and cognitive theories such as Bem's (1967) self-perception theory.

Relationship between attitudes and behaviour

The link between attitude and people's subsequent behaviour is complex and provides controversy in this particular field. Little correlation has been found between what people say their attitudes are and their overt behaviour. Researchers and theorists have gone on to develop theories to explain this complex relationship. Social psychologists attempt to provide explanations for the conflict between what people believe and the way that they behave.

Theory of Reasoned Action (Fishbein & Ajzen 1975) and Theory of Planned Behaviour (Ajzen 1988)

The theory of reasoned action was developed by Fishbien and Ajzen in the 1970s. They suggested that the best way to predict behaviour is to ask the person if they intend to participate in the behaviour.
  Their theory comprised:

- Subjective norm – what others might expect them to do
- Attitude towards behaviour
- Intended behaviour

If these are known then behaviour can be predicted. This theory was later extended and called the theory of planned behaviour. This included another element: perceived behavioural control (see Chapter 7 for further discussion of this model, and Figure 7.2).

Box 5.5   Example of theory of planned behaviour

The nurse's *attitude* towards smoking is that people should not do it, but his/her colleagues smoke (*subjective norm*). The nurse does not believe he/she has control over colleagues' behaviour (*perceived control*). Therefore his/her *behavioural intention* is not say anything to the colleagues about it. The nurse has his/her coffee break with the colleagues and sits in the smoking area with them and does not complain (*behaviour*).

  Therefore, if the researchers knew what the nurse's attitude was, what the subjective norms were, and their perceived control and behavioural intention, then they may be able to predict the nurse's behaviour.

There have been a number of theories developed to predict people's behaviour which incorporate an attitudinal element. Some of these will be explained in Chapter 7 under the heading 'Health models'.

Attitude change

If the premise is that attitudes can influence behaviour, then learning how to change someone's attitude can be important to nurses in a number of ways.

Nurses frequently need to address people's attitudes in health-related areas, for example:

- Smoking
- Eating
- Taking medication
- Safe sex
- Exercising

Nurses need to deal with people's attitudes to facilitate their becoming well, maintaining their health and improving their health; this is usually called health promotion.

It has been suggested that there are two major ways in which to change attitudes:

- Persuade the person to change their attitude.
- Persuade someone to behave counter to their attitudes in the expectation that their attitude will alter accordingly.

After World War II the United States of America's government financed a research study to explore persuasive communication, over concerns of propaganda used during the war and fears of threat in the 'cold war' period. This was called the Yale approach and was led by a researcher called Hovland (Hogg & Vaughan 1998).

Their explanations of how to change attitudes can be categorised in term of:

- Factors concerning the communicator or 'persuader'
- Factors concerning the persuasive message itself
- Factors concerning the target of the message, 'the persuadee'

They identified various factors about the message, the source or persuader and the audience or persuadee, that influenced the likelihood of changing a person's attitude and showed that the processes of attention, comprehension and acceptance were significant.

Some of their findings are, in outline:

- Experts are more persuasive.
- Popular and attractive people are more persuasive.
- Rapid speech is beneficial.
- The message is more persuasive if it is seen to be directed to someone else.
- If message induces fear it is more persuasive.
- Low self-esteem increases the chance the message will be persuasive.

- If distracted the message is more persuasive.
- When the audience is hostile it is better to offer both sides of an argument.
- Information presented first is remembered best (primacy effect).

This has come under some criticism more recently, with suggestions that people with high self-esteem and intelligence are not less persuadable but are more likely to deny being persuaded, rather than actually being protected from a persuasive message. Also, this pragmatic research offers limited explanation on why people are persuaded.

Despite this, the information that the Yale approach has collected can be useful for nurses as it can guide them in their health promotion.

Box 5.6   Example of how the Yale approach findings might be helpful to nurses

If a nurse wishes to persuade a client that they need to take more exercise to increase their well-being and reduce the risk of ill health, the nurse may consider the following:

- State the most important information first – the person needs to increase their exercise to . . . (*primacy effect*).
- Explain why they need to do this, highlighting the risks (*induce fear*).
- Ensure they have a good understanding of what the nurse is advising and why (*be an expert*).
- Ensure that the nurse has taken care of their appearance and is acceptably attractive to the person (*attraction*).
- Speak confidently.
- If the person appears hostile to the advice, then offer an understanding of how this has disadvantages as well.

Summary

This section has considered what constitutes an attitude, how it is formed and what function attitudes perform. It continued by considering the relationship between attitudes and behaviour, and finally explored attitude change.

Stereotyping and prejudice

It is also important that nurses are aware that attitudes are not all neutral or benign, and that people can hold both positive and negative attitudes. Whilst positive attitudes are said to be enhancing to well-being, negative attitudes can lead to prejudice and discrimination.

Stereotyping is defined as a 'widely shared and simplified evaluative image of a social group and its members' (Hogg & Vaughan 1998, p. 312). Gross (2001) suggests that this occurs through the following process:

- A person is assigned to a particular group (such as black, gifted or disabled).
- It is believed that all members of this group share certain characteristics (the stereotype).
- It is believed that this individual has these characteristics.

There has been debate in recent years as to whether stereotyping is useful or problematic. It was suggested that placing individuals in stereotyped groups did not allow for individual differences as no two people in a group are exactly the same. More recently it has been recognised that stereotyping also provides a useful purpose; it allows people to make, sometimes necessary, quick judgements, and reduces the work toll on the limited cognitive capacity.

Box 5.7   Example of stereotyping

One of the people you are caring for you know has epilepsy and they are about to enter the television lounge where a programme with flashing lights is showing. You quickly make a judgement based on the stereotype that flashing lights can trigger an epileptic fit in people who have epilepsy. Due to this stereotyped judgement you quickly intervene to stop them entering the room. Although flashing lights might not be a problem for this individual, the stereotype has enabled you to protect their well-being.

Although it has been recognised that stereotyping can be useful to the nurse, allowing them to make quick judgements, it can also create problems when these pre-judgements or prejudices lead to discrimination.

> **Box 5.8 Example of discrimination**
>
> If you refused to allow the person with epilepsy to watch the television in the lounge at all because there might be a programme on that showed flashing lights, this could be seen as restricting their freedom due to a stereotype and would be discriminatory.

Nurses frequently need to deal with issues of stigmatism and prejudice occurring towards the people with whom they work. Stigma refers to a person with a visible sign that they belong to a certain group or are outside of the dominant group. There are many groups within society who experience prejudice and discrimination, including:

- Certain racial or religious groups
- Physical deformity, disease or amputation
- Mental illness or disability
- Homosexuality
- Certain occupations

Given that nurses work with all racial and religious groups, occupations and sexuality, they will need to consider issues of discrimination that may be expressed towards the people they are caring for, as stated in their code of conduct (NMC 2004). It is also crucial given that their patients or clients may be doubly discriminated against due to experiencing more than one of the above, for example they may be nursing a person with a facial disfigurement who is homosexual.

Prejudice and discrimination is an area that documentary makers are particularly fond of and 'unfairness' or lack of equity in health provision is frequently a target due to its emotive nature. There have been numerous programmes that have highlighted the plight of older people, obese people, people who smoke and those with mental health problems. These programmes have helped people to recognise prejudice. With this enhanced recognition the government has instigated initiatives such as the National Service Frameworks (DoH 1998) and the National Health Service Plan (DoH 2000). Through these and other initiatives, effort has been put into reducing health inequalities, but given the finite nature of health funding difficult decisions will continue to need to be made. Some of these judgements may continue to be based on stereotyped prejudices, such as older people have had most of their lives so younger people should be given certain treatments.

Rungapadiachy (1999) suggests that attitudes and prejudice are two of the main influencing factors guiding nursing care. He goes on to say that understanding patients' or clients' attitudes can help nurses see the situation from their perspective and establish why they behave in the way they do. For nurses it is important that they are aware of their attitudes, particularly their prejudices, despite the difficulty in changing them, as an awareness can assist the nurse in not acting on them and behaving in a discriminatory manner.

Section summary

This section of the chapter has considered what attitudes are, how they are formed and what functions they perform. The relationship between attitudes and behaviour has been explored, along with attitude change. Finally, stereotyping, stigma, prejudice and discrimination have been considered.

Groups

Definitions

Hogg and Vaughan (1998, p. 234) define a group as 'two or more people who share a common definition and evaluation of themselves and behave in accordance with such a definition'.

Carlson et al. (2004, p. 659) define a group as 'a collection of individuals who have a shared definition of who they are and what they should think, feel and do – people in the same group generally have common interests and goals'.

Groups are important to nursing and healthcare as most nurses work as part of a team, either intraprofessional – the nursing team – or interprofessional or multi-disciplinary teams, where nurses work with other health professionals such as doctors, occupational therapists, physiotherapists and social workers. The government, in numerous publications, have stressed the importance of healthcare professionals working together to enhance the care given and the well-being of the people being cared for.

Baron and Byrne (1991) list the criteria that an aggregate of people need to possess to be an effective group:

1. Interact: Members of the group must interact with each other.
2. Interdependent: The implication that what happens to one member affects all others.
3. Stable: The relationship must last for a significant length of time (weeks, months, years).
4. Shared goals: Some goals must be common to all members.

5. Structure: Structure allows each member of the group to have a set role.
6. Perception: Members must perceive themselves as being part of a group.

Group formation

Many theories and models exist which explain the process of the development and maintenance of groups. It is suggested that a life-cycle approach is useful in the understanding of groups and that groups go through set stages in the process of development and maturation.

Stages in group life, developed by Tuckman (1965):

- Forming
- Storming
- Norming
- Performing

Rungapadiachy (1999, p. 174) lists a fifth stage, adjourning/mourning, where once the group task has been completed, the group disbands and becomes a social group.

Case study   Developing a team approach to Clara's care

Nurses work within a variety of teams, some of them intraprofessional and some interprofessional.

Clara has complex health needs and is living in the community, but needs a group of healthcare professionals to care for her. She has had learning difficulties throughout her life but has managed, with support, to initially maintain paid employment and more recently manage her relationship with her partner, who also has a learning difficulty, and their two children. Clara has had a stroke (CVA) but had become quite distressed while in hospital so her rehabilitation is continuing at home. She needs support with her personal hygiene, mobility and housework, including cooking and childcare. Her husband needs to continue to attend his paid employment. On her discharge from hospital, her nurse organises who will be part of the team to care for Clara, with the multi-disciplinary team. The team comprises an adult nurse, a learning disability nurse, a physiotherapist, an occupational therapist, a doctor and a social worker. They meet with Clara to organise a plan of care.

Initially they spend some time discussing how to plan the care and are led by Clara and the nurse with whom she has already formed a relationship on the ward (*forming*). After a couple of weeks meeting twice a week as a whole team, they review the care and there is quite a lot of animated discussion about the best methods of responding to Clara's needs, with some suggesting that Clara would be best served by going back into hospital (*storming*). A revised plan is eventually agreed on and the care continued. At the next planned review the team carefully discusses Clara's care and health status; a number of options to develop the care are considered and the care plan reviewed (*norming*). The care continues smoothly for a few months, with regular reviews and adjustments (*performing*).

Effective and ineffective groups

A key concept within group effectiveness is group cohesiveness. Cohesiveness can be seen as the extent to which a group hangs together; if it is cohesive it hangs together closely. Festinger et al. (1950) developed a model suggesting that a 'field of forces' influence group cohesiveness (see Figure 5.1).

Festinger et al.'s field of forces involves attractiveness of the group and its members and the mediation of goals through the interaction and interdependence of the group members. If the members find the group and its members attractive and they can work well together

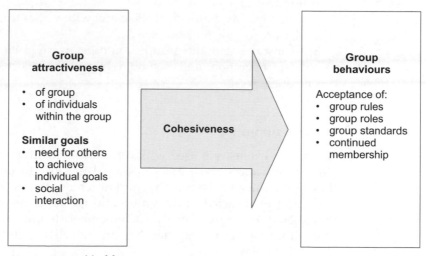

Figure 5.1 Field of forces.

with mutually dependent goals, this is the field of forces and the group will be cohesive. This cohesion will lead to behaviours such as continued membership and an acceptance of group values, roles and standards.

McGregor's (1960) work on group cohesiveness is more pragmatic. He suggests factors that influence group effectiveness, rather than a theoretical framework. He says that the following factors influence the effectiveness of groups:

1. Atmosphere: which needs to be relaxed and comfortable, free from tension, with all members interested and involved.
2. Discussion: this should be focused and with all members involved.
3. Objectives: should be clearly understood and accepted by the group members.
4. Listening: all members should listen to one another, so that everyone feels free to express himself or herself.
5. Disagreement: if there are disagreements, the group should know how to deal with them without avoidance.
6. Decisions: should be made by consensus rather than simple majority rule; the group should try to find ways to ensure consensus of all of the members.
7. Criticism: this should be kept open and members should be able to be comfortable with constructive criticism.
8. Feelings: the members should able and willing to express their feelings freely.
9. Action: should be clearly defined and all members should be fully committed to it.
10. Leadership: this should be flexible and with no domination by the leader or struggle for power.
11. Self-consciousness: the group should be aware of its modes and rules of operation, and it should frequently reflect on its own operation.

Section summary

Groups are extensively used within healthcare, with nurses being part of both intra and interprofessional groups. To be effective these groups need to be cohesive, and to achieve this each member needs to feel attracted to the group and the other members and they should have agreed goals. Each member should feel comfortable within the group and that they are an active member with a clear role to play.

Relationship theories

As can be seen by the previous parts of this chapter, the interactions between people are crucial within healthcare. Nursing care needs to be provided from within a team, which to be cohesive needs each of the group members to be attractive to each other and the group. Nurses also need to interact and develop relationships with their clients or patients. The therapeutic relationship is considered in more detail in Chapter 6, so other types of interaction are considered here.

People are said to need to have relationships with others, and if the psychological perspectives are considered it can be seen that they all recognise the importance of the interaction with others.

It is perhaps prudent to consider self through the idea of self-concept before considering the need for affiliation, liking, attraction and love.

Self-concept

Biopsychologists have a limited view of the self, which focuses on the physical body: genetics and neural and chemical effects, which influence behaviour. The biopsychologists offer biological explanations for affiliation, liking, attraction and love. Therefore their focus is on the physical elements of the self and *body image*.

Psychodynamic theorists are particularly interested in the unconscious part of the self (see Chapters 1 and 2), the part that is unknown to the individual. They seek to explore this and the unconscious forces that maintain the personality. These forces, life and death, driven along with repressed memories, are given as explanations for the person's understanding of themselves and their interactions with others.

Cognitive psychologists are interested in how people process information or think about things. These thoughts are said to influence both feeling and behaviour, including interpersonal behaviours such as liking and love. The cognitive *schema theory* (see Chapters 1 and 4) can be used to understand self-concept, as suggested by Marcia and also *Bem's self-perception theory*.

Humanistic psychologists offer quite a complex understanding of the self through the work of theorists, such as *Rogers' self-concept* (see Chapter 6) and *Kelly's personal construct theory* (1955). They suggest that each person is unique and develops towards his or her own personal potential. They therefore seek to understand attraction and love through individualistic drives or motivations.

Behavioural psychologists do not have a particular interest in individual self-concept, but within the bridging work between behavioural and cognitive theories, the work of theorists, such as Bandura's (see

Chapters 1 and 2) explanation of the development of self-concept, becomes an issue to be explored. Also, the work of social psychologists such as *Goffman's dramaturgical self* (1959) can be seen behavioural in nature.

All of these theories are useful for nurses in order to understand themselves and those with whom they work, but there are other social theories of self-concept that do not fit neatly into one of the perspectives, such as *James' social comparison* (1890) and *Cooley's looking glass self* (1902).

Body image

A person's body image allows them to recognise the difference and boundaries between themselves and others, which is necessary in a social world. According to Stewart (2005), body image is:

- The perception of one's own body, conscious or unconscious
- The picture a person has of their own body, which is formed in their mind
- The way in which a person's body appears to themselves
- One's mind's eye picture of oneself

The way in which a person views their body can have an immense impact on the person, their self-esteem, self-worth and behaviour. Body image can involve the person's perception of their height, weight and hair and their gender. Disease, dysfunction and trauma can distort a person's body image. When a person undergoes any body image changes, such as mastectomy or a skin condition, a readjustment of the person's functioning occurs. In extreme cases such as phantom pain after an amputation or a person with anorexia nervosa, sometimes this body image can differ from objective reality.

Bem's self-perception theory

Bem's self-perception theory (1967) is linked to attribution theory and opposes the cognitive dissonance theory developed by Festinger (1957). The theory of cognitive dissonance proposes that if a person observes themselves as behaving in a manner that is in opposition to their attitudes, they change their attitudes as to hold conflicting pieces of information about oneself is psychologically uncomfortable. Both cognitive dissonance and self-perception theory derive from the cognitive perspective suggesting that people process information and make decisions about themselves and others. Bem suggests that people watch themselves and decide what their attitudes are through attributing attitudes to themselves by watching their own behaviour.

Case study   Bem's self-perception theory

Julie has recently qualified as a nurse and she believes it is important to be non-judgemental to her patients and practise ethically. She finds that when a patient called Sarah comes into outpatients for treatment, she avoids being the nurse to give this treatment. After some reflection Julie realises it may be due to Sarah's sexuality. This causes Julie to feel uncomfortable with herself.

Cognitive dissonance theory would suggest that this discomfort (dissonance) would lead Julie to change her attitudes or behaviour.

  Self perception theory would suggest that using an attributional process, Julie would assess if this were something that she does with other patients that possess the same sexuality as Sarah. If Julie found she did behave in this manner with other people with this sexuality, she would conclude that she had negative attitudes towards people with Sarah's sexuality. If Julie observes herself responding differently towards other people with Sarah's sexuality, then she might attribute her behaviour towards something to do with Sarah's attitudes or behaviour.

Kelly's personal construct theory

Kelly's personal construct theory is usually considered to be based in the humanistic perspective. It recognises that each individual is unique and as they grow they learn about themselves and the world, constructing theories and testing them out like scientists. He suggests that this developed knowledge of the world is organised into constructs which can be seen as continuums with a negative and positive pole. Kelly went on to develop what he called a repertory grid through which these constructs could be explored. These have also been used in therapy to help people understand how unhelpful constructs about themselves can precipitate mental health problems.

Case study   Kelly's personal construct theory

David has approached his tutor because he does not feel he will be able to complete his course and make a good nurse. The tutor suggests that David use the repertory grid that he had been learning about in his psychology session. David chooses two other student

Continued

nurses he feels he knows well and plots a repertory grid. He initially identifies constructs that he believes they have in common and those that he believes they do not. He also identifies constructs about himself.

Constructs	David As he sees himself	David As he would like to be	Tom	Jason
Clever	No	No	Yes	Yes
Skilled	No	Yes	Yes	Yes
Confident	No	Yes	No	Yes
Caring	Yes	Yes	Yes	Yes
Friendly	Yes	Yes	Yes	No
Warm	Yes	Yes	Yes	No

Using this approach David was able to assess what it was he was trying to achieve for himself in his desire to be a nurse, and to assess, in a scientific manner, how well he was achieving this in relation to his peers. It allowed him to recognise what he thought was important in nursing and where he needed to put more effort to achieve this.

Goffman's dramaturgical theory

Goffman's dramaturgical theory (1959) suggests that a person's character is only the role they are playing at any given time. When a person is working as a nurse they take on all the behaviours of a nurse but when they leave their work environment and go home they then take on the role of a brother or sister, mother or father, etc. He suggests that there is no distinct self; people are merely the role they are playing at any given moment. Although Goffman is not a behaviourist, this theory of self-concept is probably the closest to a behavioural explanation, in that it might suggest that people have learnt to behave in certain ways in certain situations.

James's social comparison theory

James, in his social comparison theory (1890, cited Gross 2001), proposed that people make comparisons between themselves and other significant people in their lives to identify their self-concept. They compare themselves with others.

Cooley's looking glass self

Cooley's (1902) theory on self-concept was, like James's, a social theory. Unlike James, he did not suggest a direct comparison was made with others, but that individuals work out how others are judging them and from this decide what they are like. This has been called the looking glass self. The people, instead of describing what they see of themselves in the mirror or looking glass, describe what they believe others can see. This can be problematic for them as it is not easy to know what people's judgements are unless they communicate this explicitly, and people also, at times, are deceitful.

Section summary

As a start to understanding relationships, the theories of self-concept have been considered through each of the psychological perspectives and some social psychological theories. All of the psychological theories of self-concept appear to indicate that people need others in order to gain an understanding of themselves. It could be suggested that most people need to have contact with others; we are social beings. This can therefore have an impact on the well-being of an individual and their recovery from illness.

Interpersonal relationships

On first meeting, people start to form impressions and judgements about each other. These judgements influence the type of relationship that ensues. These relationships can be seen as at least partly culturally determined. Western societies place emphasis on romantic relationships between two people, but other cultures put emphasis on the extended family and responsibility.

Physical attractiveness

The first time a new person is met, the first thing that will be noticed is how physically attractive they are, and even people who meet over the World Wide Web have chosen to do so after inspecting a picture that has been posted by the other person. As with other groups of people, there is a physically attractive people's stereotype. It is assumed as part of this stereotype that the person will be warm, sociable, friendly, and successful in all areas and enjoy life. There is also evidence to support the stereotype, as physically attractive people are more likely to be offered a job at interview and likely to receive good evaluations of their skills.

Physical attractiveness is seen as partly cultural, when the bound feet of China and the elongated necks in Africa are considered, but there seems to be some consensus on facial attractiveness, with more symmetrical faces seen as more attractive. This could be explained through a biological–psychological perspective in that symmetrical faces can be indicative of good genes and development.

Proximity, familiarity, similarity and reciprocity

One theory of relationships is that proximity of another person may lead to a relationship, whereas distance may lead to relationships ceasing. Proximity offers the opportunity to get to know one another and develop a relationship, although this needs to be within the social boundaries of personal space. Personal space is the area around a person within which they feel uncomfortable if others move inside. This differs between sexes and relationship types, along with individual preferences. On the whole, personal space is culturally determined; it can be seen that Europeans who live near the Mediterranean allow others physically closer to themselves than the English. Personal space can be a particular issue for nurses, who may need to invade an individual's personal space in order to provide care. It is important that nurses explain the need to move into a person's private space and gain consent beforehand.

Despite the need to deal with personal space, psychologists suggest that socially appropriate proximity is useful for nurses, as with others, to develop relationships with both colleagues and those for whom they care.

Familiarity is seen as part of the process towards attraction and leads on from proximity. If two nurses work together, they may become familiar with each other due to recurrent exposure. Although a myth suggests 'familiarity breeds contempt', psychologists have found that, as a person becomes more familiar, they are perceived as more comfortable to be with. This understanding from social psychology is important for nurses in their relationships with their patients or clients.

Case study   Proximity and familiarity

Rosie is a community nurse. She visits Mrs Ravenhill once a week to check her progress and dress her leg ulcer. Mrs Ravenhill is 79 years old and quite frail. She is nervous of strangers and has several locks on her door. She sometimes becomes a little confused, especially on days when she has forgotten to take her medication. Rosie visited Mrs Ravenhill before she left the community hospital so that she would recognise Rosie when she called at her home. Rosie is aware that Mrs Ravenhill has gradually become more relaxed with her and now appears pleased to see her. Proximity and familiarity have allowed Rosie to develop a therapeutic relationship with Mrs Ravenhill.

Case study   Limited proximity and familiarity

Mrs Ravenhill is soon to leave hospital. She has been given a letter that tells her the name of the community nurse and when they will call, as the nurses at the community hospital are aware Mrs Ravenhill can become forgetful and confused. She is also anxious due to her frailty. The community nurse calls at Mrs Ravenhill's home and as Mrs Ravenhill is quite anxious, takes some time to explain what she needs to do, the medication and when the nurse will come again. The following week a different community nurse calls at Mrs Ravenhill's home. They too need to spend some time reassuring Mrs Ravenhill, who is slightly reticent to allow them to look at her ulcer. Eventually the nurse completes the visit but records the level of anxiety expressed by Mrs Ravenhill. As this continues, Mrs Ravenhill is prescribed extra medication for her anxiety, which exacerbates the confusion and forgetfulness. If the community team had recognised the importance of proximity and familiarity in developing an effective relationship with Mrs Ravenhill, they may have ensured a regular nurse.

Along with proximity and familiarity, similarity and reciprocity are also seen to be important in developing and maintaining relationships. If people have similar attitudes, beliefs and values, they tend to find each other more attractive. Also, people tend to like others more if they believe they are liked in return; the liking is reciprocal.

Rubin (1973, cited Gross 2001, p. 408) suggests that similarity is rewarding because:

- Agreement may provide a basis for engaging in joint activities.
- A person who agrees with us helps to increase our confidence in our opinions.
- Most people are vain enough to believe that anyone who shares their views must be sensitive and praiseworthy.

- People who agree about things that matter to them generally find it easier to communicate.
- We may assume that people with similar attitudes to ourselves will like us and so we like them (reciprocity).

Social exchange theory

This theory is based on a reward approach of operant conditioning (behavioural perspective) but goes beyond this, as it is interactional. Homans (1961, cited in Hogg & Vaughan 1998) adapted the basic operant conditioning of Skinner to incorporate some economic concepts. These concepts included:

- Cost reward ratio – working out what one has to give (cost) in a relationship in comparison to what one can get (reward).
- Minimax strategy – the concept that people try to give as little as possible for the greatest gain.
- Profit – where the rewards (what is gained) exceed the costs (what has to be given).
- Comparison level – the standard by which other relationships are judged.

Within a relationship, costs and rewards could be material, emotional, informational, services or status. This theory suggests that people are not altruistic; they are attempting to gain as much as possible and whether a relationship works is dependent on each person believing that they are gaining an appropriate reward for their efforts. More recently in western societies, there has been a focus on equity within relationships. The expectation is that there should be no profit but that each person should make the same effort and receive the same level of rewards.

Theories of love

The development and maintenance of relationships as described above account for any type of relationship. Some would suggest that different types of relationship have different meanings and therefore differing explanations are needed. Whilst the theories above may be useful to the nurse for shorter term relationships, it may be important to consider other types of relationship that a nurse may experience. There has been some discussion as to the level of relationship that should be experienced by nurses and patients in the therapeutic relationship, with some suggesting that the counselling or therapeutic relationship is more similar to a loving relationship.

Hogg and Vaughan (1998, p. 467) offer a definition of two types of love:

- *Passionate (or romantic) love* – a state of intense absorption in another person involving physiological arousal
- *Companionate love* – caring and affection for another person, which usually arises from sharing time together.

Sternberg (2000) offers a triangular theory of love, which incorporates many types of love. He suggests that love has three basic components: intimacy, passion and commitment.

- Intimacy refers to a closeness or connection with another person, within which thoughts feeling and hopes are shared.
- Passion is the desire, an intense erotic attraction, to unite with another person.
- Commitment is the intention or decision to stay within a relationship.

Sternberg's theory gives eight types of love which are dependent on whether intimacy, passion or commitment are part of the relationship:

- Non love – where there is no intimacy, passion or commitment
- Infatuated love – where there is only passion
- Liking (friendship) – where there is only intimacy
- Empty love – where there is only commitment
- Romantic love – where there is passion and intimacy
- Companionate love – where there is intimacy and commitment
- Fatuous love – where there is passion and commitment
- Consummate love – where passion, intimacy and commitment are present

Sternberg suggests that people develop their own personal love stories, and love relationships only develop when another person is found to take on the fantasised role. Both individuals need to fulfil the fantasised role of the other, and as long as they do this the relationship continues whatever type of love the story holds.

An understanding of love relationships is important for nurses and others in the caring professions, whether nurses believe that their relationships with patients or clients constitute a love relationship or not. If has been found that love relationships have a profound impact on people. Stroebe et al. (1982, cited Hogg & Vaughan 1998) identified that people who had recently been bereaved of their love partner were much more likely than other people of the same age to die. This was particularly so for the 20–29-year-old age group (10 times higher). Nurses need to ensure those bereaved have an adequate social support network, and offer time and support.

Chapter summary

This chapter initially focused on how nurses form an understanding of their own and other people's behaviour through what is known as attribution theories. These theories offered explanations of how a nurse may make judgements and predictions about the behaviour of those with whom they work. The next section explored attitudes, how these develop, their function, and how and why nurses may seek to change them. Then the psychological theories that enhance the understanding of working with individuals were considered. The chapter moved on to use psychological theory to understand how people work together as groups. Finally, the chapter ended by returning to understanding oneself in a social context, and individual relationships and love.

References

Ajzen, I. (1988) *Attitudes, Personality and Behaviour*. Milton Keynes: Open University Press.

Allport G. (1935) Attitudes. In C. Murchison (ed.) *Handbook of Social Psychology*, Vol 2, p. 810. Worcester, MA: Clark University Press.

Baron R. & Byrne D. (1991) *Social Psychology: Understanding Human Interaction*. London: Allyn and Bacon.

Bem D. (1967) Self perception: An alternative interpretation of cognitive dissonance phenomena. *Psychological Review*, 74, 183–200.

Carlson N.R., Martin G.N. & Buskist W. (2004) *Psychology*, 2nd edition. London: Pearson Education.

Cooley C.H. (1902) *Human Nature and Social Order*. New York: Scribners.

Department of Health (1998) *National Service Frameworks*. London: HMSO.

Department of Health (2000) *The NHS Plan: A Summary*. London: HMSO.

Festinger L. (1957) *A Theory of Cognitive Dissonance*. Evanston, IL: Row Peterson.

Festinger L., Schachter S. & Back, K. (1950) *Social Pressures in Informal Groups: A Study of Human Factors in Housing*. Stanford, CA: Stanford University Press.

Fishbein M. & Ajzen I. (1975) *Belief, Attitude, Intention and Behaviour*. Reading, MA: Addison Wesley.

Goffman E. (1959) *The Presentation of Self in Everyday Life*. Harmondsworth: Penguin.

Gross R. (2001) *Psychology the Science of Mind and Behaviour*, 4th edition. London: Hodder & Stoughton.

Hogg M. & Vaughan G. (1998) *Social Psychology*, 2nd edition. London: Prentice Hall.

Kelly G.A. (1955) *A Theory of Personality: The Psychology of Personal Constructs*. New York: Norton.

McGregor D. (1960) *The Human Side of Enterprise*. New York: McGraw Hill.

NMC (2004) *Code of Conduct for Nurses*. London: Nursing Midwifery Council.

Pennington D., Gillen K. & Hill P. (1999) *Social Psychology*. London: Arnold.

Rungapadiachy D. (1999) *Interpersonal Communication and Psychology for Health Care Professionals: Theory and Practice*. Oxford: Butterworth Heinemann.

Sternberg R.J. (2000) *Pathways to Psychology*, 2nd edition. London: Harcourt College Publishers.

Stewart W. (2005) *An A–Z of Counselling Theory and Practice*, p. 60. Cheltenham: Nelson Thornes.

Tuckman B. (1965) Developmental sequences in small groups. *Psychological Bulletin*. 63, 384–99.

Managing the Therapeutic Relationship

6

Learning Objectives

All nurses need to engage in relationships with those for whom they care, even if the person on whom they are focusing is unconscious. The relationships between nurses and their patients or clients are considered to be helping relationships and therefore therapeutic. Given the essential therapeutic nature of these relationships, it is important that nurses have an understanding of how to manage these to enhance the care they give.

- Discuss the differing explanations and interventions for each of the psychological perspectives in relation to the therapeutic relationship.
- Identify why self-awareness is important within the therapeutic relationship.
- Recognise the core elements of a therapeutic relationship.

Introduction

The focus of this chapter is how and why nurses might develop and utilise the therapeutic relationship. It will consider each of the psychological perspectives in term and explore what understanding they can provide the nurse. It will explain the core components of any therapeutic relationship, highlighting the relationship between these and their psychological underpinning. Examples will be given to enhance understanding of how this psychological knowledge can be applied to the nurse's clinical practice.

The term 'therapeutic relationship' is used extensively in healthcare, but what counts as a therapeutic relationship? Is this a counselling relationship or is it something more basic such as any helping relationship, which could include collecting a person's shopping? The terms 'therapeutic', 'counselling' and 'helping' relationship appear at times to be used interchangeably.

If a dictionary or thesaurus is used to examine each of these terms, it can be found that therapeutic is something to do with treatment, which may involve counselling. It is also something to do with advice and helping, and to do with enabling or assisting. Within the nurse–patient relationship the nurse could be considered to be doing all of these activities. Psychological theorists refer to the therapeutic relationship, the counselling relationship and the helping relationship, not in the eclectic manner used by many nurses, but using the terms individually, which gives each of these approaches some distinction.

This chapter will primarily use the term 'therapeutic' with the understanding that therapeutic is to do with offering appropriate treatment, whether that is offering advice, administering medication or helping with other problems. This will be explored through the relationship that the nurse has with the client or patient. The nurse–patient relationship is unique but can be supported by psychological theory.

Each of the psychological perspectives offer a different approach to managing the therapeutic relationship, but one thing that all approaches expect is that the person managing the relationship has some awareness of themselves – self-awareness.

'Self awareness means being in touch with one's thoughts, feelings and actions . . . being consciously aware of one's own existence.' (Rungapadiachy 1999, p. 282)

As discussed in Chapter 2, emotional intelligence is considered important in nursing care, and one of the five key elements of emotional intelligence is self-awareness. Literature on emotional intelligence informs us that to work well with others we need to understand and manage ourselves (see Chapter 2).

Self-awareness

The development of self-awareness is a choice but once the choice has been made it has consequences for the nurse; although some would suggest that to be a caring nurse self-awareness is essential. Once the nurse starts to develop self-understanding, they are then faced with the need to address issues about themselves.

Box 6.1   Example of self-awareness

The nurse has just read that people with depression may experience psychomotor retardation (a slowing down of their actions), and along with feeling low they may experience feelings of guilt and shame. The nurse recalls that he/she had become irritated that a person he/she was caring for was not moving away from a potentially risky situation quickly enough, and had admonished them. On reflection the nurse identifies that another approach may have been more helpful. The nurse had developed some awareness of his/her feelings and behaviour and as part of this has recognised the need for change in themselves.

Nurses develop their self-awareness through techniques such as reflective practice. The student nurse is taught models of reflection to guide them, but nurses are expected to continue to develop these skills once they become registered nurses. Reflection is also used as part of clinical supervision (see Chapter 3).

There are numerous elements that influence a nurse's behaviour and it may be useful for nurses to reflect on these to develop self-awareness. These include:

- Thoughts
- Feelings
- Behaviour
- Beliefs
- Attitudes
- Values
- Hopes and fears
- Likes and dislikes
- Past experiences

Developing self-awareness can be seen as a lifelong approach and those with greater awareness could be considered to be more mature, but chronological age is not necessarily correlated with self-awareness.

Luft and Ingham (1955) developed a model which suggests that there are four quadrants of awareness. It is called the Johari window (see Figure 6.1).

This model suggests that there are parts of ourselves that are kept private and that there are parts that can only be seen by others, but also there is a part of the self that cannot be seen by ourselves or others. This might be considered the unconscious part of the self, but only some psychological theorists accept the concept of the unconscious mind and that the self is not totally open to the person. In therapy or

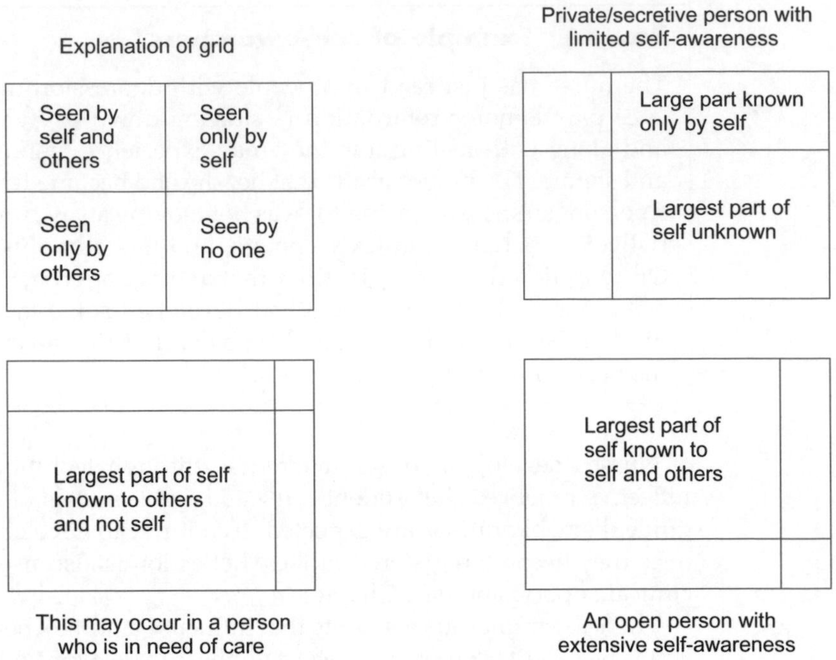

Explanation of grid

Seen by self and others	Seen only by self
Seen only by others	Seen by no one

Private/secretive person with limited self-awareness

	Large part known only by self
	Largest part of self unknown

Largest part of self known to others and not self	

This may occur in a person who is in need of care

Largest part of self known to self and others	

An open person with extensive self-awareness

Figure 6.1 A simplified version of Johari's window.

therapeutic relationships, the aim is to enable the person to be aware of their self-concept and make changes to it if they find that would facilitate their well-being. If nurses do not have a good sense of themselves, they may be seen as at best ineffective and at worst incompetent by those they are trying to help.

Psychodynamic therapeutic approach

The development of self-awareness can be traced back to the work of Freud who was particularly concerned with unconscious processes and how they influenced the experience of the present. His psychoanalytic approach to therapy involved bringing to consciousness memories the experiences that had been repressed so that they could be addressed and the person could move on – increasing their self-awareness.

Freud suggested that behaviours are guided by the three conflicting components of the mind or psyche (see Chapters 1 and 2):

- Id is the innate pleasure-seeking part of the mind, which initiates automatic responses or reflexive responses to the world. The id is located in the unconscious part of the mind.

- Ego is the rational realistic part of the mind, which manages the conflict of the other two parts of the mind. It resides in the mainly conscious part of the mind, repressing the desires of the id until an appropriate social situation occurs.
- Superego is the idealistic part of the mind and attempts to ensure behaviours are moral according to rules of parents and society. Most of the superego resides in the unconscious mind.

Freud suggested that the unconscious drives of the id are the motivating forces in a person's life; these he labelled the life drive (Eros) and death drive (Thanos). The motivating force for the life drive is libido. Freud believed that this motivation for sexual fulfilment was present at birth.

Box 6.2   Life drives and death drives

Life drives such as hunger, thirst and elimination lead to behaviours to fulfil or extinguish these drives or needs.

Death drives such as aggression, suicide and homicide lead to behaviours to extinguish these drives or needs.

These drives could motivate the behaviours of the nurse who is working with people who are vulnerable due to their health problems. It is therefore important for a nurse to be aware of these drives in themselves, to manage them effectively.

Nurses, as with other people at times, use mental defence mechanisms to deal with these drives within their social environment, to manage the inner conflict caused by not fulfilling these needs immediately (see Chapter 1). Mental defence mechanisms can resolve the unfulfilled need in the short term, but in the longer term the need must be addressed.

Psychoanalysis suggests that needs and desires unmet in childhood will affect the adult personality, and to resolve problems in the adult personality these unconscious needs or desires should be brought to conscious awareness. There are four techniques that are used to achieve this (Cave 1999):

- Free association
- Dream analysis
- Transference
- Information leakage such as parapraxes (also know as Freudian slips)

The psychoanalyst uses this information to interpret the problems for the person. Their interpretation is then given to the client to enable them to manage their lives.

Whilst nurses may not in general use psychoanalysis in managing their therapeutic relationships with clients, there are some techniques that psychoanalysis offers that might be useful.

Transference

This is where a client transfers their feeling, and sometimes consequential behaviours, about a significant person in their lives onto the analyst. The analyst may in turn, through countertransference, respond to the client as if they were a significant person in the analyst's life, such as their daughter, mother, etc. The analyst will use this information to understand and interpret the person's problems, but transference can occur in other therapeutic relationships that are not intended to be psychodyamic; they are non-analytic situations.

Box 6.3 Example of transference and countertransference

You are working with a middle-aged woman, who this morning needs assistance getting herself out of bed and washing and dressing. The woman is usually polite and grateful for the help given by nursing staff, but when you assist her she becomes agitated and defensive about her abilities, pushing you away. You respond by dropping things and accidentally breaking her hairbrush, and blaming her for the breakage saying, 'Why did you do that?'

An explanation could be that the woman is expressing *transferred* feelings, which she has placed on you. She may have been severely criticised as a child for not organising herself in the morning. This has led to her being generally overly self-deprecating and in this situation she has behaved in the way in which she would have done as a child. She has *transferred* the responses she made to her parent to you.

You, as the nurse, instead of being efficient have become clumsy and uncomfortable with the woman due to her rejection of you. This has triggered a pattern of behaviour you developed in childhood when faced with rejection. You would seek any reason to give your parent not to reject you – *countertransference*.

Information leakage such as parapraxes (also know as Freudian slips)

Information leakage can be observed in a number of ways, but one that is identified particularly in this perspective is parapraxes. Freud says that no behaviour is accidental, all behaviour has meaning, and so if a person makes a parapraxis or Freudian slip, that has meaning and is giving the therapist information about the person's concerns.

Box 6.4 Examples of parapraxes

You are doing an assessment of a client's holistic health needs and are being slightly disturbed by their smell. You intended to ask them if they regularly had their bowels open but instead asked them if they regularly had body odour.
Or
The nurse passes a breakfast tray to a young man and he responds 'thank you for the breast breakfast in ages' instead of 'thank you for the best breakfast in ages'.

There are other forms of leakage that are important to nurses and can be seen in body language or physiological changes, such as blushing. Although nurses will not be using this information to develop a deep interpretation of the client's psyche, it can still offer clues as to their problems and worries. This additional information can be used to enhance the therapeutic relationship.

There are a number of newer psychodynamic therapeutic approaches, including object relation theory developed by Klein (1882–1960), who worked with Anna Freud to develop play therapy. This is where children are observed playing and given the opportunity to transfer their thoughts and feelings about significant relationships onto the playthings and the therapist. The therapist then offers the child an age-related interpretation of their problems so that they can develop understanding and influence change.

Section summary

Although most nurses may not use a psychodynamic approach to therapy with their clients, it can offer understanding for the nurse about themselves and their clients. It also highlights the usefulness of leakage that can help guide the nurse in their relationships. An awareness of psychodynamic techniques should enhance the management of the therapeutic relationship.

Behavioural therapeutic approach

This psychological perspective has been outlined in Chapters 1 and 3. The behavioural psychologists believe that babies are born with the in-built ability to learn and that all their behaviour, including language, is learnt. The behaviourists particularly focus on the relationship between the person or animal and their environment, and see the organism learning from its environment. This learning occurs at a primitive level by habituation through to classical conditioning and then operant conditioning to social learning theory. Each of these stages can be seen as hierarchical:

1. Habituation learning by familiarisation
2. Classical conditioning learning by repetition and pairing (association and law of exercise)
3. Operant conditioning learning through reinforcement and punishment (reward)
4. Social learning theory learning by observation and imitation (vicarious)

Classical conditioning

Developed by Pavlov (1927), the main characteristics of the learning process are extinction, generalisation and discrimination. The conditioning or learning occurs when a person reflexively responds to a given stimulus. This reflexive response can be trained (conditioned) to occur with a previously unassociated stimulus. Hence this can be referred to as learning by association; if one stimulus is associated with another stimulus that produces a certain response, after a period of time both stimuli will gain the same response.

Operant conditioning

Thorndike (1913, cited Cave 1999) developed the concept of instrumental conditioning, accepting the principles of Pavlov but introducing the element of reinforcement. This development was continued by Skinner (1938, cited Cave 1999) and became operant conditioning. This approach is based on the law of effect, which states that when something good happens after an action, the behaviour is likely to be repeated. The characteristics of classical conditioning still occur (extinction, generalisation and discrimination), but behavioural shaping through successive approximation is also said to occur in operant conditioning (Cave 1999). Learning also occurs in a more explicit manner where a person will learn that to do one thing rather than another produces a reward (operant conditioning). This can be seen in many animals as well as people. Skinner suggested that in the real world animals do not just respond to one stimulus and so he looked at how they *operated* within their environments.

In operant conditioning, learning is either achieved through training by a teacher or as a matter of 'trial and error'; in either situation rewards or punishment influence the learning and future behaviour.

Both of these theories of learning can assist the nurse in their management of the therapeutic relationship. There have been a number of therapies that have developed from these two learning theories.

Therapies based on classical conditioning:

- Systematic desensitisation
- Aversion therapy
- Exposure therapy

Therapies based on operant conditioning:

- Behaviour modification
- Token economies
- Stimulus satiation

Classical conditioning

Systematic desensitisation

This approach is used with feared or anxiety-provoking situations. The assumption is that the person is fearful or anxious about an object or situation due to maladaptive learning or unhelpful associations, and so the person needs to relearn how to respond in the given situation. 'Systematic' refers to a graded introduction to the feared situation and 'desensitisation' refers to the counterbalancing or reducing of the fear response. Counterbalancing can be achieved by activities such as progressive relation or medication.

Box 6.5 Example of systematic desensitisation

A person you are working with needs to have regular blood tests but is fearful of this intervention. A graded plan of introduction (systematic) could be developed and the person taught to how use progressive relaxation (counterbalancing).

Continued

Progressive relaxation is where the person works systematically through their body, tensing and relaxing each muscle so that they develop control over their muscles and an understanding of what tensed and relaxed muscles feel like. When in a fear-provoking situation they can then counterbalance the muscle tension of the fear response with the relaxation of each muscle.

The plan could involve initially the person habituating to seeing needles by having one in a place where they frequently go. This could progress to going to sit in the chair where they would normally have their blood test. At each step the person should be allowed the time to feel in control of their fear and then move on to the next step.

Aversion therapy

This therapeutic approach is used to extinguish unwanted behaviours such as alcohol abuse or sexual deviance. Many techniques have been used to create an unpleasant response when doing the undesired behaviour. For a person abusing alcohol, medication such as antabuse (disulfiram) can be prescribed which induces a feeling of being very unwell; they become hot with flushing, feel nauseous and vomit when they drink alcohol. The antabuse is the unconditioned stimulus; the alcohol becomes the conditioned stimulus and the vomiting is the response (see Chapter 1). Electrical charges have been administered to drug addicts as an aversion to stop their drug-taking behaviour, and elastic bands have been used. The elastic band is worn around the wrist and the people 'ping' themselves if they do something they should not.

Exposure therapy

This is where the stimulus is repeatedly presented without the opportunity of response and so the behaviour becomes extinct.

Summary

For nurses, behaviourism has a lot to offer particularly in managing the therapeutic relationship. Classical conditioning demonstrates the importance of staying in a fearful situation until the fear has been extinguished, and that responses to stimuli will determine whether behaviour continues. A client could associate a nurse with an unpleasant response, or alternatively a nurse may become a conditioned stimulus to a positive response.

Box 6.6   Example of classical conditioning

A person has been in emotional discomfort, the nurse (conditioned stimulus) gives the person time to talk through their problem (unconditioned stimulus), and the emotional pain is replaced by comfort (response). The nurse becomes associated with the relief of emotional pain.

Or

A person has been in emotional distress, the nurse (conditional stimulus) tells the person they are too busy to talk to them (unconditional stimulus), and the emotional pain continues to be experienced (response). The nurse becomes associated with emotional pain.

Operant conditioning

Behaviour modification

As this therapeutic approach is based on operant conditioning, it aims to reinforce desired behaviours. Usually a behavioural plan is drawn up with clearly specified goals, baseline behaviours are established, the behavioural strategy is identified, and once the plan is in place it should be monitored and changed if necessary. This approach is used particularly with animals and children, as the desired goal or reinforcing (rewarding) small sub-goals along the way, slowly shape behaviour.

Box 6.7   Example of behavioural modification

Lovaas et al. (1967, cited Gross 2001) used a behavioural modification approach with autistic children, slowly shaping their behaviour and developing language by using food as a reinforcement.

Token economies

Again, this is using the approach of reinforcing desired behaviours; in this case a token is used to reinforce the behaviour. Most schools use this approach with the children (star charts and house points) and it has been used in psychiatric hospitals (tokens which can be redeemed at the hospital shop). It can also be seen in the use of loyalty cards in supermarkets, and modular nursing programmes collecting marks to gain an average that will lead to a good degree classification.

Stimulus satiation

This is where the reinforcement is overused, as too much of anything can become a reason for extinguishing behaviour. Too much food, too much time and too much attention can all extinguish a response.

Box 6.8   Example of satiation therapy

Azrin (1965, cited Cave 1999) explains where stimulus satiation was used to extinguish psychotic stealing of towels. The patient had been stealing towels at every opportunity and so the nurses were encouraged to offer the patient more towels and not to remove those already in her room. After a while the patient started emptying her room of towels without being asked.

Summary

The operant conditioning behavioural approach can also offer the nurse guidance in managing the therapeutic relationship. As explained in the examples above, it can be used as part of the treatment regime for clients but also as part of the underpinning relationship between nurse and client. It highlights the importance of reinforcement, especially positive reinforcement or reward which facilities the continuation of a behaviour. Nurses needs to ensure that they offer positive reinforcement to those with whom they work.

Social learning theory

Another form of learning that builds on classical and operant conditioning is social learning theory, which acknowledges a cognitive element to learning (see Chapters 1 and 3). The theory suggests that learning can occur not only by association and reward but also by observing others' behaviour and imitating it – *vicarious learning*.

Albert Bandura and colleagues developed the theory of social learning through a number of experiments; these demonstrated that observational or vicarious learning could occur. For this type of learning to take place there needs to be another person or people to learn from; this person is usually referred to as the *role model*.

Role modelling can be important as part of the therapeutic relationship. If the nurse wishes to influence a client's behaviour through their therapeutic relationships, then they could take on the task of a role model.

Effective role models

There are certain features that make a role model effective; these features enhance the vicarious learning. An effective role model possesses the following attributes:

- They are rewarded.
- They are similar enough to imitate.
- They are well thought of or respected socially.

This would suggest that for a nurse to be a good role model and to develop a therapeutic relationship, they need to be similar to their clients or patients, to be liked and appear to be rewarded. Bandura also identified that along with the concrete skills, people, especially children, also develop an understanding of their values and attitudes, along with problem solving and self-evaluation, from their social environment.

Self-efficacy

Self-efficacy is an important factor in prompting a behaviour or motivation. The social learning theory approach suggests that a person's motivation to attempt modelling behaviour is dependent on the person believing they can accomplish that behaviour. Self-efficacy is developed from previous experiences of the same or similar situation. It is important that nurses are aware of and develop their own self-efficacy and that of the people with whom they work, to achieve positive outcomes.

This can be seen within the therapeutic relationship where nurses carry out procedures that are necessary for their patients or clients. If the nurse is an effective role model for that person, the person will attempt to carry out the procedure demonstrated by the nurse. The nurse must ensure that they have the ability prior to the attempt, as failure will reduce the person's self-efficacy and reduce the nurse's effectiveness as a role model. If the nurse is unsure of success, they can break the task or procedure into small achievable chunks to facilitate success, increase self-efficacy and maintain the therapeutic relationship.

Cognitive behavioural therapeutic approach

Cognitive behavioural approaches initially developed from the behavioural perspective in psychology. The approach of Pavlov and Skinner was seen to be too mechanistic and a shift occurred through the work of psychologists such as Thorndike and Bandura, leading to the cognitive perspective.

The work of Tolman (1920s, 1930s and 1940s, cognitive behaviourism) and Bandura (1960s and 1970s, social learning theory), along with theorists such as Piaget (1930–1970s, cognitive development), led to the evolution of cognitive psychology (Gross 1996). Alongside cognitive theorists, there were others interested in therapies. They too recognised the inadequacy of a purely behavioural or psychodynamic approach. Ellis (1962, cited France & Robson 1997) provided the cognitive elements to behavioural therapy, leading to rational emotive therapy. This work continued to be led by Beck (1976, cited France & Robson 1997) and Meichenbaum (1977, cited France & Robson 1997).

There have been a number of therapies developed in this area:

- Beck (1967, cited Cave 1999), whose background was in psychoanalysis, focused on automatic negative thoughts and identified the cognitive triad leading to cognitive therapy.
- Ellis (1962, cited France & Robson 1997; 1991, cited Cave 1999), whose background was in psychoanalysis, developed rational emotive therapy, which became rational emotive behavioural therapy and established the ABC model (in this case A = activating, B = beliefs, C = consequences).
- Bandura (1969 and 1977, cited Cave 1999) developed the social learning theory, which established social behavioural therapy.
- Meichenbaum (1977, cited France & Robson 1997), whose background was in behavioural therapy, developed a therapeutic approach which is called self-instructional training.

General principles

- Cognitive activity affects behaviour.
- Cognitive activity may be monitored and altered.
- Desired behaviour change may be effected through cognitive change (Dobson 2001).

It is suggested that people perform a cognitive activity called reasoning. This is where the interaction with the world is via a process of interpretation and inference. These interpretations and inferences can become distorted but are accessible to consciousness, therefore the individual can change them. People are prone to automatic negative thoughts, which have underlying distortions, referred to by Beck as cognitive schemas. These schemas may become biased and rigid, which manipulates input to fit in with this biased or rigid view of the world (Cave 1999).

Box 6.9   Example of cognitive therapy

The person has a self-schema that they are a failure. When faced with a new task, the automatic negative thought is, 'I will not achieve this, it will be a disaster.' The nurse presents a new task as part of their recovery, which is to prepare a balanced nutritious meal for themselves. They manage to plan the meal and buy the necessary ingredients, but when cooking the meal they leave out two of the ingredients. The meal has lost none of its nutrition and had a good taste. The person's automatic negative thought is, 'I missed out two ingredients, I have failed – I am a failure.' They have focused on the negative elements instead of the positive; they have interpreted the input to fit with their biased and rigid view of themselves. The person then refuses to prepare another meal, as they are a failure for which they now have evidence.

If, as suggested by Beck, everyone is prone to automatic negative thoughts, it is important for nurses to be aware of this when developing and maintaining their therapeutic relationships. At times it may be necessary for the nurse to reframe or offer an alternative interpretation of the events, or to encourage the patient or client to do so for themselves.

Box 6.10   Example of automatic positive and negative thoughts

You are caring for a person who has been undergoing tests and it has been found that the person needs an operation to rectify the problem.

The person says, 'Oh no, I might die under the anaesthetic.' (automatic negative thought).

The person says, 'Oh, I am pleased that they have found out what is wrong and that it can be sorted out' (automatic positive thought).

Or

You are caring for a person who needs to make some lifestyle changes.

The person says, 'Oh no, I can't do that, I won't remember what to do and I will get it wrong' (automatic negative thought).

The person says, 'Oh, that will be a challenge, I will have to work at remembering so that I achieve that' (automatic positive thought).

An underlying assumption of cognitive therapy is that each person has unique experiences leading to a set of beliefs and ways of interpreting the world. People then go on to act on these beliefs and interpretations. They also collect information to support the beliefs and ways of interpreting the world already held. People actively construct their view of themselves and the world. They are constructivists.

There is an interrelationship between thoughts, feelings and behaviour that has led to therapies involving both cognitive restructuring and changing behaviours. This group of therapies is known as cognitive behavioural therapies. They use the theories of both the cognitive and behavioural perspectives. They recognise the importance of association, reinforcement, beliefs and automatic thoughts (self-talk).

Ellis proposed an ABC model of cognitive therapy where A was the activating event, B was the belief and C was the consequence.

Returning to the person who failed to prepare a nutritious meal:

A – Activating event could be the task of preparing the meal.
B – According to Ellis, beliefs can be rational or irrational; this person believed they were a failure, which could be considered irrational, whereas a belief that they were not experienced in meal preparation could be considered rational.
C – (Due to irrational belief) the emotional consequence was that the person continued to believe they were a failure and felt bad, and the behavioural consequence was that they refused to undertake the task again.

Cognitive behavioural therapy is based on developing new adaptive learning, which will address the automatic thoughts and presenting behaviours. The therapist will endeavour to use the following approaches (Hawton et al. 1989):

- Problem solving
- Dealing with the here and now, not focusing on the past
- Helping the person to bring about changes in their own lives
- Explicitly agreeing goals
- One of the goals needs to be identifying the time boundaries of therapy
- Collaborative approach

The nurse could use this approach in their therapeutic relationships to help their clients or patients, and could use the associated therapeutic strategies outlined below.

The therapeutic strategies that are used include:

- Distancing/distraction
- Challenging negative thoughts
- Challenging underlying assumptions
- Building skills, e.g. assertiveness

Cognitive behavioural therapy (CBT)

Cognitive behavioural therapists accept the underlying principles of learning developed from behaviourism, but also the developments of the cognitive perspective. Problems must be current, repetitive and recordable for their techniques to be put into practice. Treatments must have well-defined goals where progress towards these goals is monitored with the client. Past history is only useful in functional analysis and choosing a strategy. Treatment plans are individualistic and should emphasise developing positive thoughts and behaviours rather than diminishing the negative. The client needs to fully collaborate with assessment, planning and treatment as the client does the bulk of the therapeutic work, with the therapist as educator and supporter (France & Robson 1997).

Section summary

The cognitive behavioural approach has a number of techniques that could be accessed by nurses managing their therapeutic relationships, particularly when the people they are working with are feeling stressed or anxious. Stress and anxiety are common in people with health problems.

Humanistic therapeutic approach

The humanistic perspective is not just one organised theory; it is based on a number of principles from psychoanalytic and behavioural thought. It is considered to be eclectic.

Maslow called it the third force of psychology, developed after the psychoanalytic and behavioural forces (see Chapter 1).

The humanist perspective was developed in the USA in the 1950s and one of the leading proponents of this approach was Carl Ransom Rogers (1902–87). Theorists from the psychodynamic and behavioural perspectives such as Freud, Thorndike and John Dewy influenced his study and theory development. He was also influenced by his own childhood deprivation.

Underlying assumptions (Nelson-Jones 1995)

- The perceptions of clients are their own realities, and that is the only reality – or phenomenological field – this is not static; it develops over time due to experiences.
- Each person has an actualising tendency, which is the basic motivating drive. This is a positive drive, allowing the organism, person, to constructively flow towards its potential.
- People are continually undergoing an organismic valuing process – placing more value on those experiences that move them towards self-actualisation.
- Humanistic psychology has a basis in existential philosophy as well as scientific psychology.

Existential philosophy

Existential philosophy premises are that an individual is (Rungapadiachy 1999, p. 80):

- Unique
- Aware of their own experience
- Creator and controller of his/her own destiny
- Completely free to make his/her own choices
- Responsible for his/her own existence

This philosophy underpins humanistic approaches and humanistic philosophy. The humanists went on to develop their own philosophy as outlined below.

The principles of humanistic philosophy

The principles of humanistic philosophy are (Rungapadiachy 1999, p. 80):

- Each individual is the chief determinant of his or her own behaviour and experience.
- Humans are conscious agents, experiencing, deciding and freely choosing their own actions.
- Becoming or self-actualising – he or she is always in the process of becoming something different.
- It is the individual's responsibility as a free agent to realise as much of his or her potentials as possible.
- People who refuse to become have denied themselves the full possibilities of human existence.

- Human consciousness, subject feelings, moods and personal experiences are crucial because they all relate to one's existence in the world of other people.

This philosophy underpinned the theories of all the humanistic theorists, including Maslow, Berne and Rogers.

There were two main areas of Rogers' work: his exploration of the self-concept and the development of client-centred therapy (CCT). As with the psychodynamic theorists, most of the humanistic theory has developed out of work with people in distress – it has developed out of the necessity of working with people therapeutically.

For Rogers, the person or client needed to understand their own self-concept to enable them to move towards their potential or to self-actualise. For Rogers, to help people in distress, as when working with people with problems, there was a need for the therapist or counsellor to see the problem from the individual perspective.

The Rogerian self-concept is complex; it is a structure as well as a process. He recognised a distinction between the 'I' and the 'me', with the 'I' being the manner in which others see the person and the 'me' the way in which the person sees themself. He suggests that people have an understanding of both of these and this is part of their self-concept. Within this self-concept people have a sense of what they are actually like (*actual self*) and what they aspire to be (*ideal self*). The person's level of self-regard or *self-esteem* is high where actual self and ideal self are close, demonstrating the equality of experiences.

Rogers also said that the way people view themselves could be congruent or incongruent. He says that incongruent implies that the self-concept is based on *conditions of worth* rather than an *organismic valuing* process. Conditions of worth are where people are doing things to achieve positive regard from others and valuing this, and not working towards reaching their personal potential (organismic valuing process) and valuing that. *Positive regard* is necessary for a congruent self-concept, but to make this the aim of one's actions is problematic as positive regard needs to be unconditional to fulfil its purpose of supporting the person towards achieving their potential. Positive regard should not be achieved through what the person does but should be given unconditionally for who the person is. Despite the problems of actively seeking positive regard, the person, through a process of *subception* and *defence*, protects incongruence and prevents change (Rogers 1951). They offer explanations and rationales for why it is important to do things to please others and gain positive regard from them.

For nurses to work therapeutically with patients or clients, Rogers would suggest they need to be congruent and have a high level of self-esteem, be positively regarded and value experiences that allow them to reach their potential.

> ## Case study Therapeutic use of Rogerian self-concept theory
>
> You are working with a woman who gained a good education. She is 30 years old and is married with three children all of school age. She spends her time organising and managing the children, the home and her husband as well as both sets of parents. She has a chronic bowel disorder and low mood (*actual self*). When talking to her about health problems you explore her lifestyle choices with her. She says she feels she has no choices as her husband, parents and children need her to continue as she is. She says she would feel too guilty to go to college or find a more fulfilling occupation (*defence*). She also says that although they do not show it, they appreciate what she is doing for them all (seeking *positive regard*). You ask her what she would be doing ideally; she says she would be a doctor and says she would have all the answers to everyone's health problems and be beautiful and glamorous with a smile (*ideal self*).
>
> This woman can be seen to be working towards gaining positive regard from others rather than accessing an organismic valuing process where she would value things that enabled her to reach her potential. Her actual and ideal self is quite distant, resulting in low mood and ongoing health problems. Her ideal self may be unrealistic but working with her to allow her to gain a realistic understanding of her potential and enabling her to work towards this, should improve her well-being. The nurse would offer the woman a therapeutic space, using the necessary core Rogerian conditions, where she can start to think about who she is and who she can be.

There are four core conditions in humanistic approaches to therapy and these are (Stewart 2005, p. 108):

- Empathy
- Genuineness or congruence
- Warmth
- Unconditional positive regard

Empathy

This is the ability of the nurse or therapist to understand the patient's or client's feelings and be able at least to demonstrate to the patient or client that they understand. It is the ability to step inside the life world of the other person, to perceive the world as they do, and to sense, feel and understand the personal meanings of their experience.

'Empathy is to feel "with". Sympathy is to feel "like". Pity is to feel "for" '
(Stewart 2005, p. 108)

Genuineness or congruence

This is to do with not adopting a role with the patients or clients with whom nurses or therapists work, but to be real. It is not behaving in a certain way because it is believed that is the way that nurses should behave, but behaving in a way that the individual nurse feels is right. It is being honest and open and not developing artificial boundaries and barriers. In a Rogerian sense, to be congruent is to have a good self-esteem, with the individual's perceived actual self and ideal self similar, which is achieved through an organismic valuing process. They should not be so distant that it causes the nurse or therapist a problem. In most therapeutic approaches the therapist is expected to be able to manage their own life.

Warmth

Warmth is displayed by the way in which people communicate. Body language and the way in which the nurse uses verbal language, as well as the words said, can demonstrate warmth. This enables the relationship to develop through a feeling of comfort and it can encourage trust. Rogers identifies a possessive and non-possessive warmth; where possessiveness is false and makes the person uncomfortable, it can be smothering. Non-possessive warmth is genuine and not demanding.

Box 6.11   Examples of how a nurse can demonstrate warmth

- Touch – shaking hands on meeting or touching arms when in conversation or holding hands if the person is anxious
- Smiling and gaining eye contact
- Using the person's preferred name
- Laughing at funny incidents described by the patient or client

The warmth needs to be felt by the nurse and once the nurse feels comfortable with showing this warmth, they can demonstrate it to those for whom they care.

Unconditional positive regard

This is the fundamental attitude that the therapist or nurse needs to adopt when working with people using this approach. The nurse or therapist needs to see and feel positive towards the client or patient, regardless of any antagonism that may be felt towards them. This is the core need for people. People have psychological problems because they have not received this in childhood and therefore cannot have a positive self-regard. The nurse needs to be accepting consistently of the person demonstrating warmth. This does not mean the nurse should be accepting of any behaviours exhibited; it is an acceptance of the person, not a particular behaviour. Nurses at times need to make clear that certain behaviours are unacceptable but that they have a positive regard for the person.

Nelson-Jones sums up the Rogerian approach with this quote:

'It is as though he/she listened and such listening as his/hers enfolds us in a silence in which at last we begin to hear what we are meant to be.'
(Lao-Tse, cited Nelson-Jones 1995, p. 40)

Summary

The Rogerian approach to the therapeutic relationship is focused on the relationship, whereas cognitive and behavioural approaches focus on the therapy or skills. The Rogerian client-centred therapy has become the basis for communication education in the caring professions, including nursing.

Gerard Egan's skilled helper

Gerard Egan, a professor of psychology and organisation at Loyola University of Chicago, developed a model of skilled helping; this is a three-stage model. Egan's therapeutic approach is from within the humanistic approach but he, unlike Rogers, recognised the need for some boundaries and goal setting within the counselling relationship and chose to call his approach skilled helping.

Egan's three-stage model involves the characteristics of a therapeutic relationship identified by Rogers, which could be considered to be:

- Respect for clients, offering positive regard
- Genuineness, congruency, trust, sincerity and honesty

- Good listening, attending and responding skills
- Empathy
- Non-judgemental approach

Egan's three-stage model of helping (Egan 1977)

1. Review the current scenario
2. Develop the preferred scenario
3. Formulation of action plans

Review the current scenario

This stage is where the helper or nurse enables the client to tell and clarify their story, which is done within the therapeutic environment felt necessary by Rogers. The helper, with the client, identifies and challenges blind spots; this is where clients are made aware of issues within their story that they had not seen. It allows them a wider perception of the problems they are trying to overcome. It is the time when the helper challenges the client to own their problems and opportunities, and to state problems as solvable and maybe faulty interpretations. The helper will also enable the client to search for leverage, which is a searching for a reason, and that to spend time and energy on the problem is necessary. If there is no leverage there is no reason to deal with the problem. Lastly, at this stage the client is facilitated to identify the complexity of the problems and prioritise them.

Developing the desired scenario

At this stage is the development of what the client sees as the preferred scenario or possibilities. It is felt important that a helping relationship has a goal, a recognised end-sight that is trying to be achieved. This preferred scenario or situation or possibilities are then changed into viable objectives or goals. Commitment to change to achieve these possibilities needs to be demonstrated by the client.

Formulation of action plans

From the identified goals or objectives an action plan needs to be drawn up. The helper and client may achieve this through a number of processes that may include brainstorming strategies for action, divergent thinking and thinking creatively. These plans need to have sub-goals with activities arranged and contingency plans if things do not happen as planned. Also at this stage, the skilled helper will need to ensure that adequate support and motivating elements are available. Egan also says that there is the need for evaluation and feedback throughout the process, to ensure success.

Box 6.12   Use of Egan's three-stage model

A person on your nursing caseload has approached you because they are having problems with their accommodation and believe it is having a negative effect on their health.

Review the current scenario
You listen attentively to what they are saying and maybe take notes; you encourage them to explain the detail of the situation and challenge their blind spots (perhaps there is something they are doing that makes the accommodation problematic). You explore with them how important it is to change the situation, encouraging them to express the problem in a manner of 'this is the way I see . . .' 'I interpret this behaviour to mean . . .'.

Desired scenario
You encourage the person to explain what they would like the situation to be realistically and get them to consider what alternatives may be available to them. Once they have considered the alternatives and identified what their preferred scenario is, you need to check that they are committed to the time and effort needed to achieve this change.

Formulation of action plans
If the desired scenario is to change where they live, sub-goals will need to be established to achieve this, and social support will need to be sought. This may need some brainstorming or creative thing to ensure that all the issues that may occur have been considered. Sub-goals, goals and contingency plans will need to be recorded to facilitate motivation and evaluation.

Summary

We have considered how the Rogerian approach to the therapeutic relationship can be formalised into a structured approach to helping people. This view of the therapeutic relationship and the helping model can be extremely useful to nurses in their therapeutic relationships with patients and clients.

The skills of helping within the therapeutic relationship

The skills of developing and maintaining a therapeutic relationship in nursing, given psychological theory and research, appear to be a caring, skilful and knowledgeable communicator. The nurse appears to need to be educated and knowledgeable about people and how they respond; the nurse needs to be self-aware not only of their external behaviours but also of their internal motivations and desires. Most importantly, they appear to need to genuinely care about the people with whom they work.

Whilst so far this chapter has considered the psychological theory of why a certain approach should be taken, fundamental to all of these approaches is the ability to:

- Listen
- Attend
- Respond

If a nurse is unable to do these then he or she will be unable to develop a therapeutic relationship based on trust.

Egan (1977) offers a basic format for listening and attending:

S – sit squarely; this means sitting upright and alert
O – open posture; crossing arms and legs may appear to be a barrier protecting the nurse from the client
L – lean forward; how far forward will depend on what is being said. If the client is distressed, leaning forward could be a sign of concern; but if the person is agitated or anxious, it may feel like an invasion of their space
E – eye contact; a consistent gaze is important but should not be constant as this could indicate disapproval
R – relax; if the nurse appears relaxed and confident, this will influence the feeling of the client and they may feel reassured

Egan (1977) also offers nurses information on how to respond within their helping or therapeutic relationships.

Verbal responding could include the following techniques:

- The appropriate use of questions that are open (for encouraging the person to talk) and closed (such as when the person is confused or in pain and information is needed).
- Reflecting (demonstrating empathetic understanding by inwardly digesting what they have said and offering it back to them in a different verbal format).

- Paraphrasing (a brief response using the person's own words may condense the information).
- Echoing (stating the last sentence that the person has said to encourage further explanation).
- Summarising (offering a shortened version of what has been said, including the main points).

Techniques for non-verbal responding could include:

- Postural echoing (taking up the same posture as the patient or client).
- Nodding (to demonstrate agreement and that what has been said has been heard and accepted).
- Smiling (to demonstrate warmth and encouragement).
- Touch (this is dependent on the person's need for personal space, but holding hands or touching forearms can demonstrate empathy).
- Silence (sometimes the use of silence can be helpful to allow the person time to reflect but know you are still present and attending).

The impact of the therapeutic relationship

An effective performance of the therapeutic relationship not only allows the nurse to assess, plan, implement and evaluate nursing care, but can also enhance patient or client recovery through patient satisfaction (Ogden 2000).

Patient satisfaction is regularly being monitored in health services due to the belief that patient satisfaction improves recovery rates and compliance with treatments. Ley (1988, cited Ogden 2000) developed a model of compliance through his extensive research (see Chapter 3 and Figure 3.1). This model demonstrated the interaction of memory, understanding and patient satisfaction in the outcome of compliance. Ley found that if people could remember the treatment and understand why and how to use it, and they were satisfied with the consultation with the health professional, they would comply with the treatment regime. People were satisfied with the consultation if they felt emotionally understood and supported (affective), they were given an adequate explanation (behavioural) and they felt that the health professional appeared competent. All of these issues have been addressed when exploring the therapeutic relationship.

The effective therapeutic relationship

Stewart (2005, p. 65) says that the therapeutic relationship is influenced by:

- How the nurse demonstrates the core conditions of empathy, genuineness, non-possessive warmth and unconditional positive regard.
- The client's or patient's feelings towards the nurse, which are influenced by trust, feeling safe and having faith in the nurse.
- The style of interaction of both nurse and patient or client (which could be cognitive, behavioural, psychodynamic or humanistic).
- The way transference and countertransference are acknowledged and worked through.

Stewart can be seen to have an eclectic approach to the therapeutic relationship, accepting elements from differing perspectives. In clinical practice nurses may find the same approach most useful. For the nurse to address the influencing factors above, they will initially need to develop self-awareness.

Chapter summary

To return to Johari's window, to increase self-awareness there is the need to trust others and disclose something of oneself. This allows others to offer and receive objective feedback, which in turn increases self-awareness. To effectively manage the therapeutic relationship, the nurse needs to develop self-awareness, but this is not a one-off event; it is an ongoing lifelong process much as nurses are expected to have a lifelong approach to their learning in general.

References

Cave S. (1999) *Therapeutic Approaches in Psychology. A Typical Development and Abnormal Behaviour.* Modular Psychology Series. London: Routledge.

Dobson K.S. (2001) *Handbook of Cognitive Behavioural Therapies,* 2nd edition, p. 4. New York: The Guilford Press.

Egan G. (1977) *The Skilled Helper.* Monterey, CA: Brooks/Cole.

France R. & Robson M. (1997) *Cognitive Behavioural Therapy in Primary Care, A Practical Guide.* London: Jessica Kingsley Publishers.

Gross R. (1996) *Psychology: The Science of Mind and Behaviour,* 3rd edition. London: Hodder & Stoughton.

Gross R. (2001) *Psychology: The Science of Mind and Behaviour,* 4th edition. London: Hodder & Stoughton.

Hawton K., Sakovskis P.M., Kirk J. & Clark D.M. (eds) (1989) *Cognitive Behaviour Therapy for Psychiatric Problems, A Practical Guide.* Oxford: Oxford University Press.

Luft J. & Ingham H. (1955) Johari Window, A graphic model of interpersonal awareness. In Luft J. (1969) *Of Human Interaction*. Palo Alto, CA: National Press.

Nelson-Jones, R. (1995) *The Theory and Practice of Counselling*, 2nd edition. London: Cassell.

Ogden J. (2000) *Health Psychology: A Textbook*, 2nd edition. Milton Keynes: Open University.

Pavlov I.P. (1927) *Conditioned Reflexes*. Oxford: Oxford University Press.

Rungapadiachy D. (1999) *Interpersonal Communication and Psychology for Health Care Professionals: Theory and Practice*. Oxford: Butterworth Heinemann.

Rogers C.R. (1951) *Client Centred Therapy*. London: Constable.

Stewart W. (2005) *An A–Z of Counselling Theory and Practice*, 4th edition. Cheltenham: Nelson Thornes.

How do People Cope with Suffering?

Introduction

This chapter will focus on understanding one of the major concerns for nurses – suffering. It will consider what constitutes suffering and how people cope with it. This is one of the main focuses of health psychology research, therefore an understanding of health psychology theories and research will be useful to the nurse.

The chapter will initially outline what health psychology is and the understanding it offers nurses, through the major health models and psychoneuroimmunology to a consideration of two specific case studies.

What is suffering?

Suffering is not a concept widely explored by traditional psychological texts, unlike concepts such as pain and grief. Some religious and philosophical writers focus on suffering, such as Buddhists who suggest all people suffer and therefore all deserve compassion.

Suffering appears to relate to pain, illness and disease, but people also appear to suffer in all areas of the person: psychologically, physically, socially and spiritually. Nurses need to be aware of any suffering that those they care for are experiencing, as suffering can have a profound effect on health and illness.

Ferrell (1996) offers a definition of suffering as 'a lived experience that is unique to each person'. She suggests that this experience involves the whole person and some element of threat or loss; it is an evaluation rather than a sensation or perception. Ferrell went on to consider the relationship between those caring for people who suffer and the sufferer, with a focus on nurses. She found that nurses' understanding of suffering developed with experience; their initial identification came from the 'medical model' in that patients as part of their condition experienced suffering, but she suggested that this became unsatisfying. She said that the nurses went on to identify suffering as a human experience, with the recognition of its individuality and how it touched families and friends. This was not the final stage in the development of the nurses' understanding of suffering. They ultimately felt the suffering of those they cared for themselves; it became a personal experience for the nurses. Given Ferrell's suggestion that nurses who have a mature understanding of suffering experience the suffering of those they care for, it is imperative that nurses not only develop an understanding of how the people they are caring for cope, but also of strategies that they themselves can use.

The concept of suffering will be further explored throughout the chapter, but the next step is to explore the research and models that can help nurses understand health behaviours, including dealing with suffering.

Health psychology

Health psychology is a new discipline (Roberts et al. 2001), with the British Psychological Society (the professional body for psychologists in Britain) only accepting it as a separate section within the Society in the late 1990s. This means that the boundaries are still being developed and formalised. Morrison and Bennett (2006) suggest that this is leading to four areas of health psychology developing in parallel (clinical, public, community and critical). Despite this, there is a common theme or approach taken by health psychologists in their acknowledgement that the biomedical model is insufficient for explaining health issues. Ogden (2000) outlines the approach taken by health psychologists as a biopsychosocial model:

- Bio – biological aspects of health and illness, such as viruses, bacteria and lesions
- Psycho – psychological aspects of health and illness, including behaviour and beliefs
- Social – sociological aspects of health and illness, such as class and ethnicity
- Model – referring to a framework or structure

Basically, as Morrison and Bennett (2006, pp. 29 and 30) state, health psychology is 'the study of health and illness and healthcare practices (personal and professional)'. Its aim is to:

'understand, explain and ideally predict health and illness behaviour in order that effective interventions can be developed to reduce the physical and emotional costs of risky behaviour.'

Assumptions in health psychology

There are some assumptions made by health psychologists that are useful for the nurse to be aware of. Despite the claim that their approach is more holistic than the biomedical model of health, they utilise quite a cognitive behavioural approach to people. They see human beings as rational information processors and that individuals have some responsibility for their health through their health behaviours. Their more holistic approach means that they also recognise psychological factors influencing the onset, progression and recovery from illness. Health psychologists also recommend that treatment be directed at the whole person.

Case study   A holistic understanding of ill health

You share nursing accommodation with three other student nurses. One of them, Sam, has a bad cold and a few days later you find

Continued

that you too experience headache, sore throat and difficulty controlling your temperature, and are coughing and sneezing. Despite this your other two housemates show no symptoms of illness.

A biomedical explanation could be that you have become infected with a virus that Sam had been infected with. There are a number of ways in which you could have contracted this virus: it could have been through direct contact (touching their skin etc.) or it could be through airborne particles propelled when Sam coughed or sneezed. Your immune system has not been in contact with this virus before and so it has a vigorous response, producing the symptoms you are experiencing. The treatment is to reduce the discomfort of the symptoms while your immune system fights the infection.

A biopsychosocial explanation for your symptoms of a bad cold may involve those of the biomedical model, but would also be interested in psychological and social issues that may have been influential in the functioning of your immune system, such as:

- Stress level – due to shift pattern, assignments due in, your mood, etc.
- Social issues – relationships with others at the university or nursing team, cramped accommodation due to low income, low income leading to poor nutrition, etc.

When psychological and social issues are taken into account, a more robust explanation for your other two housemates not also having symptoms is achieved. This explanation could also lead to treatment including ensuring a balanced diet, a break from shifts and a problem-solving assignment schedule, which may reduce the likelihood of becoming ill again.

Historical perspective

Hippocrates, in the fifth century BC, concentrated on identifying specific physical causes for illness. Although recognising the importance of spiritual energy, he identified that an imbalance of the four humours (blood, phlegm, black bile and yellow bile) would lead to ill health. Some of these terms are still referred to today; some people are said to be phlegmatic, meaning they have too much phlegm, which is exhibited as sluggishness and coolness.

Galen in the second century AD could be considered the next major figure in the development of western medicine. He used concoctions of various herbs and other substances to treat ill health, but he also recognised the impact of the psyche. He identified that melancholic women were more likely to develop cancer. This could be understood to mean that if a woman's mood is low, her immune system may not function well and cancer-forming cells would not be eliminated. It is suggested that this is the earliest western record of the impact of the psyche on immunity.

The middle of the sixteenth century was considered to be the birth of scientific thinking as it is now understood, although there are some who would argue with this as the early Egyptians and Greeks could be described as scientific. Despite this emergence of the scientific approach to medicine, treatment still mostly involved the alteration of the humours through herbal remedies.

In the middle of the seventeenth century Thomas Sydenham suggested that medical training should involve patients and not solely consist of scholarly activity such as the study of ancient Greek and Latin. He was also believed to distinguished symptoms from underlying causes of illness.

During this period René Descartes proposed that mind and body were different entities. This continues to have a huge impact on health services today, with mind disorders treated by psychiatrists and nerve disorders treated by neurologists.

Through the eighteenth and nineteenth centuries this reductionism progressed, with the biomedical model of health and illness becoming predominant in western societies. Over the last 30–40 years, with the increase in immune disorders and a certain amount of mistrust of medical therapies, there has been a resurgence of mind–body research and treatment. Alongside this mind–body research, there has been the development of nursing as a unique profession, with the introduction of Project 2000 in 1990 and the development of health psychology, both of which ascribe to an holistic approach to dealing with health and illness.

Premises of mind–body medicine

Holistic approaches to health have led to the development of mind–body medicine, which sets out a different philosophy of care or treatment in contrast to the biomedical approach. The premises of mind–body medicine are (Watkins 1997):

1. Mind and body are simply two aspects of a whole individual.
2. Every person has self-healing abilities.
3. Each person is unique and must be responded to as such.
4. Each person is an integration of physical, psychological, intellectual and spiritual aspects.

5. Patients' healing abilities are strongly affected by expectations and beliefs.
6. Mainline medicine does not have a monopoly on the search for health.
7. Patients need to be actively involved in their own healing and in the decision-making concerning their treatments.

Box 7.1 Example of holistic explanation of illness

As nurses are aware:

'Cancer cells grow because of the conditions favourable to them, such as toxic substances, malnutrition, genetic factors, and immune suppression. Whether or not the immune system is at fault when cancer develops, it now seems certain that bolstering the immune system can help fight malignancy.' (Watkins 1997, p. 100)

Watkins goes on to ask:

'If a woman smokes to relieve the stress of a miserable marriage, what is the cause of her lung cancer? A genetic predisposition? The history of oat-cell carcinoma? The smoking itself? Her relationship? How thorough is her cure if she has a lung removed but does not change her marital circumstances, let alone enquire into the personality patterns that permitted her to cling to her long time unhappiness?' (Watkins 1997, p. 100)

Nurses, through their holistic approach to care, are expected to take all of the woman's needs into account when assessing, planning, implementing and evaluating her care. Therefore the care for this woman may involve the lung removal mentioned and chemotherapy, but may also involve health promotion activities such as support with cessation of smoking and relationship counselling.

The premises of mind–body medicine appear to be accepted by both the holistic models of nursing and health psychologists. Researchers, including health psychologists, continue to explore the holistic nature of health and well-being, and as part of this research explore the links between the elements of the body. One of these areas has been labelled psychoneuroimmunology, an awareness of which could be very useful to nurses to support their holistic care.

Psychoneuroimmunology

Psychoneuroimmunology has been an area of prolific study since the late 1970s. Through these studies health psychologists have accepted that the nervous system, immune system and psychological processes interact. The nervous and endocrine systems send chemical messages, in the form of neurotransmitters and hormones, to each other. These chemical messengers can increase or decrease immune function, and cells of the immune system produce chemicals that feed information back to the brain. A person's emotions have been recognised as having an impact on the nervous system, and vice versa, for many years but it is only this more recent research that has implicated the immune system as well. To gain an understanding of this complex research area nurses need to have at least a basic understanding of the underpinning biology of the nervous and immune system, as well as an overview of the psychological processes involved. Later in the chapter this will be applied to two case studies.

The nervous system

The nervous system is made up of a number of components.

The central nervous system is the part that is encased by bone and includes the brain and spinal cord.

The peripheral nervous system is the part that is outside of the brain and spinal cord but includes nerves that are attached to them. It has two divisions: the somatic system and autonomic system.

The somatic system is the part of the peripheral nervous system that controls the movement of skeletal muscles or transmits somatosensory information (information about the body – muscles etc.) to the central nervous system.

The autonomic system is the part of the peripheral system that controls the vegetative functions – the internal glands and organs that the individual has little or no conscious control over. The autonomic system has two divisions as well: the sympathetic and parasympathetic divisions (Carlson 1998).

The sympathetic division is the portion of the autonomic nervous system that controls functions that accompany arousal and expenditure of energy. It can (Gross 2001, p. 61):

- Dilate pupils
- Inhibit salivation
- Accelerate breathing

- Increase heartbeat
- Inhibit digestion
- Stimulate secretion of adrenaline and noradrenaline
- Inhibit bladder contraction

The parasympathetic division is the portion of the autonomic nervous system that controls functions that occur during a relaxed state. It can (Gross 2001, p. 61):

- Constrict pupils
- Stimulate salivation
- Slow breathing
- Slow heartbeat
- Stimulate digestion
- Contract the bladder

The sympathetic and parasympathetic divisions are both controlled by the hypothalamus, which is situated in the forebrain, and within the limbic system. The hypothalamus controls these divisions of the peripheral nervous system to regulate homeostasis (balance of the physical body). The hypothalamus controls them directly by nerve impulses and by stimulating the release of hormones from the endocrine system (such as adrenaline).

The immune system

The immune system is complex and involves a number of components. This makes assessing the function of the immune system very difficult. Some experimenters have counted the level of white cells in the blood and others have used symptoms of illness, but neither of these offer a precise indication of function.

The immune system includes:

- Physical barriers such as the skin
- Mechanical barriers (coughs etc.)
- Chemical barriers (saliva etc.)
- Harmless pathogens (bacteria in nose etc.)
- Lymph nodes (tonsils etc.)
- Phagocytes – neutrophils and macrophages (when in the blood known as white blood cells but found in the lymphatic system too)
- Lymphocytes (when in the blood known as white blood cells but found in the lymphatic system too)

White blood cells

There are a number of cells that are labelled white blood cells and they each have slightly different actions. Essentially their main aim is to rid the body of pathogens; these are things that enter the body and that the immune system believes will harm the body. Pathogens could be bacteria, viruses or foreign objects. The white blood cells aim to rid the body of these pathogens. Pathogens have unique proteins on their surface called antigens, which are recognised by the immune system and stimulate it to action. Both phagocytes and lymphocytes are identified as white blood cells.

Phagocytes

- Neutrophils – short lived
- Macrophages – long lived

Lymphocytes

- B lymphocytes mediate humoral immunity
  - These cells produce proteins called antibodies that destroy antigens or enhance the ability of other cells to destroy them.
- T lymphocytes mediate cell immunity. These T cells can produce:
  - 'Helper T cells', which help enhance the ability of antibodies by the production of interleukins and lymphokines
  - 'Killer T cells', which attack antigens especially those causing tumours
  - 'Suppressor T cells', which suppress the humoral immunity.

There is also a third type of immune response cell in the blood and these are called natural killer (NK) cells; they dispose of infected or malfunctioning cells.

Psychological processes

There are numerous psychological processes that may influence health, well-being, illness and recovery, and are all studied by health psychologists:

- Perception
- Emotion and motivation
- Consciousness

- Language
- Memory
- Intelligence
- Problem solving
- Abnormal development and function
- Social cognition, behaviour and skills

Some of these will be explored in more detail in the case studies later in the chapter.

Research in psychoneuroimmunology

There has been a lot of recent research in this area due to concerns over health issues such as HIV developing to AIDS, and rates of cancer.

Impact of psychology on the immune system

There have been numerous studies undertaken to consider the impact of psychological processes on the immune system, as this is thought to be one of the major ways in which the person's psychological state has an impact on their physical health.

Many studies have looked at the presence of NK cell activity (reduced NK cell activity suggests a reduced immune response), and found that people recently bereaved or suffering from stress had lower levels of NK cell activity.

Impact of the nervous system on the immune system

Bone marrow and thymus, where immune cells develop, are well supplied with sympathetic, parasympathetic and non-adrenergic non-cholinergic nerves, and therefore they have an impact on how and when immune cells are developed. The autonomic nerves are capable of regulating almost all the cells involved in the inflammation process, which is a significant part of the immune response. Autonomic nerves, also, through a complex system of chemical release (neuropeptide, nitric oxide and polypeptides), innervate lymphoid tissue.

Section summary

This part of the chapter has considered the development of research in psychoneuroimmunology and offered a brief overview of the systems and processes involved. Whilst this offers the nurse some

---

understanding of the elements involved in the experience of suffering, it offers only a limited understanding of how this experience may be reduced, ameliorated or coped with. The next section considers health models that may assist in the facilitation of changes in health behaviour.

Health models

A health model is a structured framework for examining a given phenomenon in health. Naidoo and Wills (2001) suggest that health models are 'abstract representations of real circumstances that assist critical thinking and analysis'.

Health models have been used as a framework for research, predicting health behaviour, and as an attempt to understand responses to ill health. There are a number of health models ranging from quite simplistic to complex.

Health beliefs model

This model has its origins in the 1960s through the work of Rosenstock and was further developed by Becker and colleagues into the 1970s and 1980s. This model was developed to explore and predict a person's health behaviour. As can be seen in Figure 7.1, the health beliefs model is composed of:

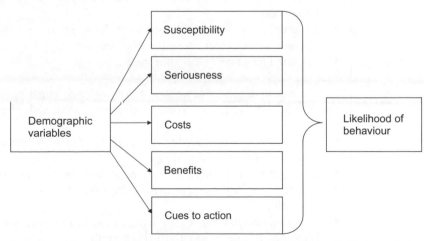

Reproduced from Ogden, *Health Psychology, A Textbook*, © 2004, with kind permission of the Open University Press.

Figure 7.1 Health beliefs model.

- Cues to action leading to perceived threat
- Perceived susceptibility
- Perceived severity
- Perceived costs and benefits

Case study   Using a health beliefs model to understand Tracey's behaviour

You are caring for a woman called Tracey. She is 40 years old, is several stone overweight and smokes. She has a family history of angina and heart attack, with her father dying at 57 due to a heart attack. You are concerned about Tracey due to her risk factors for heart problems.

When you first see Tracey at the well woman clinic, you discuss with her the possible genetic and lifestyle risks to her health. She says she does not believe she is particularly at risk as her father was male. She goes on to say she has many friends who are much older than herself who smoke and it is not a problem for them, and anyway if she stopped smoking it would increase her stress which would increase her risk of heart problems. Tracey also says she does not believe her weight is any of your business.

- *Cues to action – perceived threat* – Tracey does not believe she is at risk.
- *Perceived susceptibility* – Tracey does not believe she is susceptible.
- *Perceived severity* – Tracey does believe that heart problems can be severe.
- *Perceived cost and benefits* – Tracey does not believe behaviour change would offer more benefits than cost.
- *Predicted behaviour* – no change.

Two weeks later Tracey starts to experience chest pains, which are diagnosed as angina. Tracey's perceptions of risk change:

- *Cues to action – perceived threat* – pain is a cue to action and her perceived threat is now high.
- *Perceived susceptibility* – Tracey now sees herself as susceptible.
- *Perceived severity* – Tracey is now frightened of dying young like her father.
- *Perceived benefits and costs* – Tracey now believes that the cost of lifestyle change is less than the benefits.
- *Predicted behaviour* – behaviour change in line with health recommendations.

As can be seen from the example, the health belief model could be useful in exploring health behaviour but it has been extensively criticised. It is individualistic and does not account for the social context; it is too rationalistic and offers no room for emotional elements. This model, whilst still being worked on by its creators, has been adapted into a model called the protection motivation theory by Rogers in the 1980s.

The protection motivation theory

This model of health behaviours, like the health belief model (HBM), accepts that perceived severity and susceptibility are important for predicting behaviour, but Rogers also included the elements of response effectiveness, self-efficacy and fear. If people felt themselves to be at risk of a disease (susceptibility, fear and severity), and they had the ability to do something about this risk (response effectiveness and self-efficacy), they would be likely to change their behaviour. The difference between this model and HBM is an assessment of ability to make effective changes to risk. Although this model has addressed some of the problems with HBM, it still attracts criticism, as although it identified the intention to change behaviour, it did not identify when behaviour change would occur.

Theory of planned behaviour

The theory of planned behaviour (TPB), created by Ajzen and colleagues in the 1980s, developed out of the theory of reasoned action by Fishbein and Ajzen in the 1970s (Ajzen 1988). These models allowed for social cognition in behavioural intentions.

As can be seen in Figure 7.2, there are three major components influencing the person's behavioural intention. These are attitudes

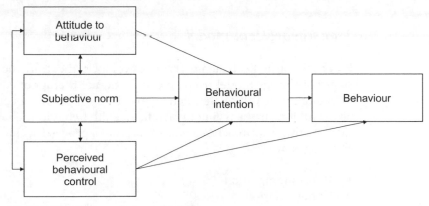

Figure 7.2 Theory of planned behaviour.

towards the behaviour, subjective norms and their perception of control over their behaviour. This is also said to have a direct impact on behaviour.

Case study   Using the theory of planned behaviour to help Rosie

You are caring for a young woman called Rosie. She has had problems accessing education owing to her dysphasia and dyspraxia. This has an impact on her self-confidence. Despite these problems Rosie recently raised the alarm when she noticed from the beach a young person in the sea who appeared to be in distress. The school that the young person attended has asked Rosie to come and tell her story and receive an award as part of a beach safety awareness day.

Rosie's *attitude* towards the request (behaviour) is that she believes she will look foolish and no one will listen to her.

Rosie's *subjective norms* are mixed as she wants to comply with other people's wishes and she knows that her friends and family will be proud of her if she gives the talk.

Rosie does not believe she is able to *control* her speech and body enough to give the talk and she feels that the environment in which she is to give the talk is uncontrollable.

This leads to Rosie's *behavioural intention* not to give the talk.

As the nurse, using this model of planned behaviour can offer you guidance on how you can support Rosie with what she believes will be an important achievement. You could explore the environmental issues with her by taking her to see the classroom prior to the talk and discuss with her and the teacher chairing the talk the likely response of the children. This may influence change in attitudes towards the behaviour and her sense of behavioural control.

Transtheoretical model

Prochaska and Diclemente (1984) developed the transtheoretical or stages of change model from an exploration of therapeutic approaches to changing health-related behaviour. This model has been found to be useful for nurses trying to facilitate health behaviour changes. Considering these approaches it was found that a process of change occurs. The stages are:

- Pre-contemplation
- Contemplation
- Preparation

- Action
- Maintenance

People do not proceed through these stages in a linear fashion, although they could. A person could jump from pre-contemplation to preparation or from contemplation to action or action back to pre-contemplation.

Case study   Using the transtheoretical model to care for Martin

You are a mental health nurse working with Martin, who has an addiction to alcohol. He has been admitted to the local mental health unit following a suicide attempt. He has been referred to your team as it is believed that his low mood, which precipitated the suicide attempt, was due in part to his using alcohol as a coping strategy for a stressful life. Since admission Martin's mood has lifted; he is no longer feeling suicidal and is ready for discharge from the unit.

You visit Martin in the unit, introduce yourself and explain why you have come to see him. Martin's response is that he does not have a problem with alcohol and so there is no need for you to spend any time with him. He assures you that he will not be drinking any alcohol when he returns home; he has got over his bad patch and is now OK. You give Martin your card and say he is welcome to contact you if he feels he needs some support in the future with alcohol use. Martin is in a *pre-contemplative stage* – he does not believe he has a problem.

Two months later Martin's GP refers him to your team again as he is aware you have had contact previously and he believes Martin is again at risk. You send Martin an appointment to see you in outpatients. Martin attends the appointment a few minutes late. This time Martin says that his partner has noticed that he is drinking too much and he is again feeling stressed and unmotivated at work. You discuss with Martin his alcohol consumption and both you and Martin agree that it is at a concerning level. Martin agrees to keep a diary of his drinking and identify the pros and cons of his consumption, and you make another appointment. *Martin is now in the contemplative stage* – he is thinking about whether he has a problem and how important it is for him to hold onto this coping strategy.

Over a number of months working with Martin he moves on to the *preparation stage*, where he is making plans for changing his

Continued

alcohol consumption and for strategies with which he can replace it. From preparation he moves into *action*, where he stops drinking and attends a support group, but over the months Martin moves from the action stage back to pre-contemplation. He then, with support, moves between pre-contemplation and action for some time, but eventually moves on to *maintenance* of abstaining from drinking alcohol.

Health action process approach

Schwarzer developed this health model in 1992 to consider health behaviours; he developed it through an extensive search through the available literature and it takes into account the features of the previous models. He identified that any health behaviour should be considered a process, or occurring in stages, not just a one-decision activity. Schwarzer proposed that there were at least two stages in the process: motivational and volition stages. As such, the use of the model attempts to predict not only behavioural intention but also behavioural action. Despite these stages, Schwarzer states that self-efficacy is the most significant factor in determining intention and behaviour.

The motivational stage is made up of:

- Risk perception   'this is a serious problem and it might effect me'
- Outcome expectancies   'if I change my behaviours I can improve my chances'
- Self-efficacy   'I have the ability to make the necessary changes'

This leads to a behavioural intention as seen in the HBM and TPB. Schwarzer suggests that once the intention to change has been initiated, the person passes on to the volitional stage. This stage, according to Schwarzer, is determined by a person's self-efficacy – initiative self-efficacy, maintenance self-efficacy and recovery self-efficacy – to create action plans and control.

Areas of self-efficacy in volitional stage:

- Initiative   'I believe I can put my plan for tomorrow into action'
- Maintenance   'It is difficult to keep going with this plan but I will do it'
- Recovery   'I did not keep to all the plan but I will, I am going to achieve this'

Schwarzer also recognised that it is not only the individual cognition and motivation that influence behaviour and behaviour change; there may also be other barriers. Perceived barriers, whether external or internal, can halt behaviour change.

Section summary

This section of the chapter has considered the health belief model, the theory of planned behaviour, the transtheoretical model and the health action process approach. The final model described has been built out of the previous models and other models and literature. Health models can be useful tools for nurses in both clinical practice, health promotion and their research, but they have not been found to be accurate predictors of behaviour, although perceived susceptibility and self-efficacy have been found to be most useful. Models like the transtheoretical are used extensively in some areas of nursing practice, such as addictive behaviours and health promotion. Health models can offer some guidance to nurses in their attempts to reduce suffering.

Personality and health

It is widely believed that a person's personality dictates whether they become ill, how they cope with illness and whether they recover from that illness. The popular press graphically presents people who fight disease such as cancer and win and those who give in to illness and die. This appears to suggest that if a person becomes ill or dies it is in some way their fault, despite a general view that people have distinct personalities at birth (see Chapter 2). Whether as a nurse you accept a genetic or biological view of personality or a learning or behavioural view of personality, there is research available which considers the impact personality has on health and illness and suffering.

A number of studies have been conducted which have identified a type A personality; people with this personality type are said to be prone to cardiovascular diseases (Morrison & Bennett 2006).

Type A personality

Researchers studying people who had had a coronary heart disease in the 1960s and 1970s identified a personality type they labelled type A personality. They identified that there were common elements manifested in people with this health problem. They were (Morrison & Bennett 2006, p. 344):

- Competitive
- Time-urgent
- Easily aroused to hostility or anger
- Impatient
- Achievement orientated
- Had a vigorous speech pattern

Type B personality

Type B personality was constructed as an opposite to type A personality, and these people were considered to be more philosophical and less at risk of coronary heart disease. Later research has been inconsistent in upholding this finding, but this may in part be due to methodological differences in the studies. However, recent research has found a more consistent link between hostility and anger and negative health outcomes.

Type C personality

A similar approach to that used in developing the type A personality has been conducted with people who have diagnosed cancer. The personality type identified has been labelled type C personality, or the cancer prone personality. People with this personality type are said to be (Morrison & Bennett 2006, p. 348):

- Co-operative and appeasing
- Compliant and passive
- Stoic
- Unassertive and self-sacrificing
- Tendency to inhibit negative emotions, particularly anger

Section summary

Despite the oversimplification of using just three or four personality types, a type D personality demonstrating negative emotions or affect was developed. There are some useful findings for the nurse working with people who are suffering. The aggressive or hostile approach of the type A personality and the passive helplessness of the type C personality coping strategy are unhelpful in people trying to recover from ill health. It would appear that neither an overexpression of emotion nor an underexpression of emotions is health inducing. This clearly links with psychoneuroimmunology, demonstrating emotions or psychological processes having an impact on the nervous and immune systems.

So far in this chapter the interaction of a person's biology and psychology have been identified, then health models were considered where it was recognised that self-efficacy and perceived control were important for people in managing their health. This section has considered the impact of personality and identified that emotional responsiveness also plays an important part in the experience of suffering.

Suffering

To return to the focus of this chapter, it can be seen that suffering is a complex phenomenon involving an intricate balance between the physiological system, such as the nervous and endocrine system, and psychological processing; it also has a sociological component.

Pain case study

The community nurse, Marie, with whom you are on placement has been asked to visit an elderly lady by the lady's GP (general practitioner). Marie has been a friendly and supportive mentor and encouraged you to ask questions if there is anything you do not understand. The GP has organised this referral for Mrs Daisy Harding, a 74-year-old widow. Mrs Harding lives independently and suffers from osteoarthritis, for which the GP has been treating her for several years. For the first few years Mrs Harding was treated with paracetamol and this was changed to co-codamol two years ago, but due to increasing pain she has been prescribed ibuprofen for the last four months. The GP believes the increase in pain is due to the progression of the arthritis, but more recently her two daughters have raised concerns about the lady's ability to cope. The family was particularly concerned as, due to the pain, Mrs Harding was no longer attending her social group at the local social services day centre, which she had enjoyed. When you both arrive at the lady's house, Marie introduces both of you and asks the lady how she would like to be addressed. The lady says that although most people call her Mrs Harding she would feel more comfortable if you called her Daisy.

Daisy offers you both a cup of tea, which you accept. Whilst she is making the tea you notice that she struggles with her mobility; she shuffles and holds herself quite rigid. When making the tea she struggles to reach the cups and teapot, as they seem to be hidden at the back of the cupboards. After she has put the tea in the pot she wraps it up in a tea towel and puts it behind the bread bin.

Daisy after a little time eventually sits with you both, drinking her tea. Marie explains why the doctor has asked you to visit and asks if Daisy would like to explain any problems she is having. Daisy explains that she has been experiencing a great deal of pain recently and it does not make any difference how she sits or lies. She says the tablets do not seem to be working. She also talks about people trying to break into her house and the loud music played late at night by her neighbours, which has bothered her. She said it is very difficult getting to sleep with the pain, worry and noise. Marie listens carefully and makes notes; she then goes on to ask Daisy questions about her general health, conducting an holistic nursing assessment including diet, exercise and mood.

When back at the health centre, Marie expresses her concern about Daisy as continual pain may increase her health problems and decrease her quality of life. Marie guides you to consider how, as nurses, you can reduce Daisy's suffering. She asks you what Daisy might mean when she says she is in pain, why you think Daisy is in pain and why it may have increased recently. You spend some time exploring these questions from the literature and find the following.

Two main types of pain

- *Acute pain*, which lasts for under six months
  - Usually relates to specific damage
  - Self-limiting
  - Disappears after repair
- *Chronic pain*, which lasts for over six months and can be benign or progressive; it does not decrease with time or treatment. It is also pain that does not diminish when the injury or disease has gone.

These timescales are fairly arbitrary but are a useful guide.

The definition of pain is partly dependent on the explanation of how it is generated. If an early explanation of pain is used, which recognises pain as a sensation, it could be defined as:

'Pain is an unpleasant sensory and emotional experience associated with actual or potential tissue damage or described in terms of such damage.' (International Association for the Study of Pain, cited Gross 2001, p. 168)

For health psychologists this definition is too limited. They suggest that pain is more than a sensation; it is a perception and although the above definition offers a psychological element – emotions – they believe there is a more complex psychological interaction occurring.

'Pain has been one of the more mysterious and elusive aspects of illness and its treatment. It is fundamentally a psychological experience and the degree to which it is felt and how incapacitating it is depends in a large part on how it is interpreted.' (Taylor 1995)

Given that research suggests that pain has a psychological element, you go on to search for an explanation for the experience of pain. In the 1960s Melzack and Wall suggested that pain is not just perceived through sensory input but can also be influenced by the person's cognitive, emotional and motivational state.

Melzack and Wall (1982) developed the gate control theory of pain, which allowed not only for biological explanations and interventions but also for psychological explanations and interventions. They accepted the idea that pain was a perception, which means that the individual is actively involved in the recognition of pain, not a passive recipient. This also allows for the recognition of multiple causes and individual variability in pain experiences.

Melzack and Wall offered an explanation of biological functioning as well as psychological functioning. They suggested the gate is situated in the spinal column. This gate is then opened and closed by biological and psychological factors.

Melzack and Wall suggest that the person receives information related to pain in two major ways: through nociceptors that transmit information about pain through the nervous system from the area of pain to the brain, and through psychological processes such as what is thought about the injury or disease (cognition) and the emotional response such as fear, anxiety, etc. So there is information being conveyed up the spinal column to the brain and information being sent from the brain down the spinal column to the area of concern.

In this situation it could be the injury that has been caused which triggers nociceptors, which open the gate to pain experience. At the same time the person knows that the injury is necessary and they are prepared for it and so their anxiety is low and they relax themselves, which could close the gate. The gate control theory includes an explanation of how the neurological and psychological processes interact through the different nerves recognising their differing speeds of action: the substantia gelatinosa, the limbic system, hypothalamus, thalamus and release of endorphins (see Figure 7.3).

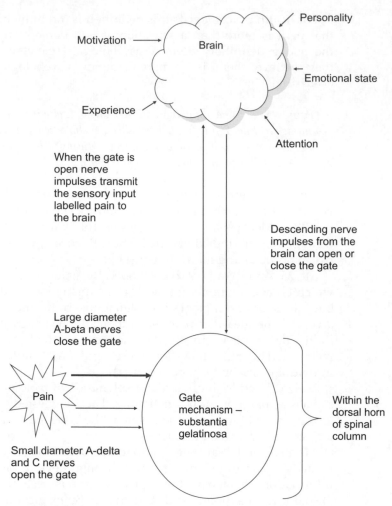

Figure 7.3 Gate control theory.

Evaluation of understanding so far with mentor

Marie is very pleased with your developing understanding of Daisy's health problems as you have identified that pain may be a perception, which can be influenced by psychosocial factors. Given this understanding it could be assumed that the increase in Daisy's pain might be due to factors other than progression of her arthritis. It could be influenced by her anxiety over people trying to break into her house, loss of pleasurable social contact and lack of sleep due to noisy neighbours. Marie asks you to consider what else might have an impact on

Daisy's pain, given the available literature on osteoarthritis, and you identify the following:

- Daisy's understanding of her problem and its treatment
- Daisy's anxiety
- Daisy's weight and the amount of exercise she undertakes
- Daisy's social support and coping strategies

With your increased understanding of Daisy's health problems, Marie supports you in explaining your understanding to Daisy's GP. The GP says they are happy to reconsider the medication regime if you can help Daisy to manage her pain. Marie then leads you to consider your approach with Daisy, and you both develop an action/care plan.

This is written using knowledge of Melzack and Wall's gate control theory of pain, psychoneuroimmunology and health models. These allow you to recognise, when organising Daisy's care, that psychological, biological and social areas of Daisy's life are all important. If you address all areas you have maximised your opportunities for enhancing Daisy's well-being. The health models also highlight the importance of self-efficacy and perceived control when seeking to change people's health behaviours.

Initial care plan

- To discuss Daisy's diagnosis with her, providing her with the information you have collected.
- To discuss Daisy's nutritional needs with the dietician and pass this information on to Daisy.
- To facilitate Daisy's attendance at the day centre so that she can gain support from others with similar problems and can access physiotherapy and occupational therapy support.
- To use a problem-solving approach with Daisy to deal with people breaking in and noisy neighbours.
- To identify Daisy's coping strategies and how these can be developed.

Marie agrees that this approach offers a biopsychosocial package of care for Daisy.

Biological/physical

- Medication
- Weight – nutrition and diet
- Exercise
- Occupational needs such as aids

Psychological

- Self-efficacy – through information giving, developing skills (coping) and offering support
- Positive cognitions – through role modelling and problem solving
- Emotion – addressing issues of concern

Social

- Addressing issues with neighbours and local community
- Offering a regular social event and contact with others
- Offering social support

Implementation of planned care

Marie organises for you both to visit Daisy again, to negotiate with her your planned approach to her care. You discuss with Daisy the elements that you have learnt are important to reduce her pain and increase her quality of life.

Daisy is fearful of some of suggestions as she feels in too much pain, so your first approach is to develop a relationship with her and develop her understanding of her health problem. As part of this you explore what strategies she uses to cope with her pain at the moment and you get a more detailed account of the problems with neighbours and burglars. It becomes apparent that as Daisy is in pain she is more alert to any noises and it has been the creaking of her outside gate that has led her to believe there are burglars. You organise with Daisy to keep a diary of disturbing noises and to discuss this with her daughters when they visit.

The next time you visit, Daisy meets you smiling. She says she wrote down the noise problems and showed her daughters and they had the outside door hinges oiled and the latch fixed so it now stays shut. They had also spoken to her neighbours who had no idea their music was causing her problems, and the neighbours had also agreed to watch out for any signs of people attempting to break in. Daisy says her sleep has improved. You spend time with Daisy discussing her diet, her ability to care for herself at home and her coping strategies for pain.

Daisy agrees to try to make changes to her diet informed by the information provided by the dietician, but still feels unable to attend the day centre yet. As Daisy continues to struggle in her kitchen, you agree with Daisy to ask the occupational therapist to do a kitchen assessment with her.

Marie reassures you and Daisy that reducing her stress, her weight and getting some sleep will all help with the pain relief. Marie encourages you to explore further approaches to coping that could help Daisy and you find that both psychological and nursing texts offer similar suggestions.

You discuss with Daisy her pain experience and it becomes apparent that at certain times of the day she feels the pain worst; these are when she gets up in the morning, after she has been sitting for a while and in the evening at bedtime. Daisy explains the only way she tries to cope with this is to try to ignore it and take tablets. You explain to Daisy that there are a number of ways she could cope with the pain experienced.

- Relaxation techniques
- Guided imagination
- Distraction
- Complementary therapies such as aromatherapy
- Activities

At the next meeting you and Marie have with Daisy she explains that she told her daughters about your suggestions and they bought her a relaxation tape to listen to at night and some lavender water to go on her pillow. Daisy says she feels as if she has more energy and is now ready to go to the day centre again, especially if they will be able to give some more suggestions. Daisy says although she is still in a lot of pain she is hoping that the next time she sees the doctor she might be able to reduce her tablets.

Evaluation

Marie, your mentor, was extremely pleased with your ability to develop your understanding of the patient's health problems, using the biopsychosocial model which allowed you to support Daisy as she developed her ability (self-efficacy) to cope and to organise her own support, both professionally and socially. Marie pointed out that Daisy's pain experience was obviously having a huge impact on her quality of life, leading her to feel quite depressed. Now Daisy feels more able to cope, her anxiety has decreased and her mood has lifted, allowing her to move more freely and feel less pain.

Stress case study

One of the clients in a residential care home, Mike, who you have been caring for, has recently been discharged from a short admission to a big acute hospital following an operation to remove a small lump from his bowel. The lump was found to be benign and there was no need for follow-up care. Mike is 46 years old, has learning difficulties and suffers from panic attacks. Any change in Mike's daily routine triggers a panic attack, but despite these problems Mike had continued to work in a nearby factory. He is now considered to be fit to return to work but is spending most of his day in bed feeling unable to tidy his room or cook for himself. You feel very concerned about this as Mike was always friendly and helpful and seemed to get enjoyment out of his employment.

Mike says he is too ill to get out of bed; he says that as soon as he gets up he feels dizzy and as if he is going to vomit. He is also complaining that his heart is racing and he cannot breathe; he recognises this is similar to having a panic attack, when he feels as if his heart is going to stop and he will die, but this goes on and on. He therefore believes that there is something very wrong with his health but people are not telling him what this is.

You explain your concerns to the interprofessional team so that a new care plan can be devised for Mike.

The assessment and treatment options are discussed and the team chooses to take the biopsychosocial approach to Mike's problems as they recognise that physical, psychological and social elements all impact on a person's health and well-being.

Physical examination found that Mike's blood pressure and pulse are higher than normal but his temperature is within normal boundaries, and blood tests identified a slightly high white blood cell count. It was decided this may be due to his recent operation, but it should be reviewed the following week.

The cognitive assessment found that Mike was dwelling on his health and interpreting any bodily function as a sign of ill health. Mike believed that he had cancer but no one was telling him, and that he would die soon. He also believed that if he stayed in bed and looked after himself, he would live longer.

Emotionally Mike was feeling anxious and low in mood and that he was a hopeless case; he became quite distressed when encouraged to perform any activity.

Socially Mike was avoiding others by remaining in his room; he was not happy for the other residents to come into his room to see him and he was refusing to return to work. Mike had also regularly attended the local church but he said he was too ill to go at the moment.

The team decides that Mike is having acute anxiety problems due to increased stress related to his recent physical health problems.

Definitions of stress

Stress is where the demands of a situation exceed the personal and situational resources to cope with it' (Roberts et al. 2001). This seems to correspond with general assumptions about stress, although some might suggest that it is the perceived personal and situational resources, not the available resources, that lead to stressful experiences.

Selye's General Adaptation Syndrome (1956)

There are a number of models of stress that allow a conceptualisation of the experience. In 1956 Selye developed the general adaptation syndrome (GAS), which offered a process of a person experiencing stress.

Using this model it can be seen that in Mike's situation, once he realised he had a physical health problem (*perceived stressor*), he went into the *alarm reaction*. This is actioned in the sympathetic branch of the autonomic nervous system (ANS). The release of neurotransmitters, such as noradrenaline and stress hormone, was triggered, having an immense impact on the physiological state of the person. At this stage the person is said to be in the 'flight or fight' syndrome, where the body is being prepared to run away or face the problem. If the person has not been able to use any of the energy being released to fight or run, the person goes into the *resistance stage*. This is where the body starts to recover, with reduced ANS activity, but as the stressor remains there continues to be an increased output from the adrenal cortex of cortico-steriods. For Mike, despite the lump being removed, the stressor has remained as he continued to believe he was at risk of dying. The next stage if the stressor has not been removed is *exhaustion* where the excitation of the ANS continues but the body's resources are becoming low. The adrenal glands do not function well, blood glucose level drops and disorders that may be of a cardiovascular nature or cancer may occur (see the section on psychoneuroimmunology earlier in this chapter). So Mike's fears may become a self-fulfilling prophecy.

Physical outcomes of prolonged stress

When a perception of stress is made, as indicated in GAS, a physiological response is initiated. There are two main systems involved in this and they are particularly of interest to psychoneuroimmunologists. These systems offer a physiological explanation for the negative impact of stress on health and how psychological processes, neurology and immunology are interrelated. The two systems are the sympathetic (relating to the sympathetic nervous system) adrenomedullary (referring to part of the adrenal glands) system (SAM), and the hypothalamic-pituitary-adrenal (HPA) axis. Although SAM and HPA are seen as separate systems, it is more useful to accept them as a united response to stress. If a stressor's existence is momentary, the HPA may not be triggered but SAM will be as it is almost instantaneous (Evans et al. 2000).

The HPA system involves a stressor, perceived possibly through the sensory organs, which is mostly relayed through the thalamus via nerve impulses/neurotransmission. This information is sent to the hypothalmus, which can trigger the release of hormones and neurotransmitters. The hypothalamus activates the pituitary gland with corticotrophin releasing factor. The pituitary gland secretes adrenocorticotropic hormone (ACTH); this activates the adrenal glands, particularly the adrenal cortex, which in turn release corticosteriods. Corticosteriods can have a profound effect on the body's immune system, as has been identified in cases of HIV and AIDS progression (Evans et al. 2000). They also reduce the inflammatory process and increase metabolism of sugars and proteins.

SAM is closely linked to the HPA when a stressor is recognised and the hypothalamus stimulates the locus coeruleus (LC) nodules (two small nodules on either side of the brain stem) by releasing corticotropin releasing factor (CRF). The locus coeruleus also stimulates the hypothalamus in return, by releasing noradrenaline (NA), and both hypothalamus and locus coeruleus and behaviour are influenced by the serotonin present. The NA from the LC, the CRF released from the hypothalamus and the serotonin all influence the behaviour of the person. Other elements of the SAM are the medulla part of the adrenal glands, which produce adrenaline and noradrenaline; these innervate tissues through the sympathetic nervous system and produce the symptoms of stress or anxiety (Evans et al. 2000). Some of the short-term symptoms of stress can be faster heartbeat (palpitations), 'butterflies' in the stomach, tense muscles and sweaty hands. Some of the symptoms of long-term stress are headaches, muscle aches, indigestion, high blood pressure, heart disease and loss of appetite.

Cognitive phenomenological model of stress (Lazarus 1966)

In the 1960s Lazarus considered the idea that thoughts, emotions and situational demands had an impact on the stress experience and coping. Over the years Lazarus and his colleagues refined this model and in 1991 Folkman and Lazarus described the cognitive phenomenological transactional model of stress and coping (see Figure 7.4).

This can offer a complementary understanding, along with the physiological impact and GAS of Mike's situation.

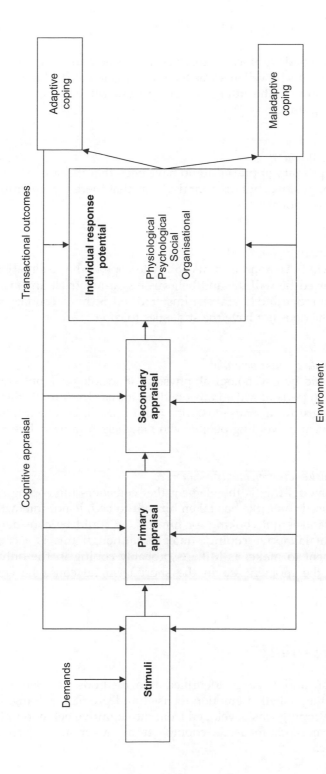

Adapted from Bailey R. & Clarke M. (1989) *Stress and Coping in Nursing*. London: Chapman and Hall.

Figure 7.4 Cognitive phenomerological transaction model of stress.

Stressor
Mike has had significant stressors in that he had symptoms of problems with his bowel, this was then investigated and a lump was found and removed. The lump was benign but Mike is having difficulty accepting this.

Primary appraisal
Mike's primary appraisal could have been that the situation was irrelevant or positive, but his appraisal was that there is something wrong and it is serious.

Secondary appraisal
Mike will have appraised his ability to cope with the situation and as he believed he will die and believes he cannot trust anyone, he feels unable to cope and has taken himself to bed. So his secondary appraisal is that he does not have the strategies to cope.

Individual response potential
This could be psychological, physical or sociological, but varies from person to person. Mike is responding to his stress in all the areas he is feeling unwell, nauseous, dizzy and low; he is catastrophising his situation and avoiding people who may help him to feel better.

Individual environmental consequences
In the model this is the element that considers the coping strategies being used. As Mike has taken himself to bed, is not interacting with others and is not cooking for himself, he could be considered to be using maladaptive coping strategies; although this is a contentious judgement to make, as Mike is probably coping in the only way he can at the moment, so in the short term he could be considered adaptive.

Coping strategies

Folkman and Lazarus identified two methods of adaptive coping, which they labelled emotion-focused and problem-solving. Problem-solving coping was developed from the cognitive behavioural theories and emotional-focused coping from a more psychodynamic approach.

Problem-solving coping

As was seen in Chapter 3, where nurses' learning was considered, the behavioural theorists offered an approach to maximise learning. This approach can be applied to coping. It involves breaking down the problem into smaller chunks so that the problem appears to be more easily overcome as it is approached one sub-goal at a time. These sub-goals should be small and achievable and when successfully completed some reward should be gained. Considering alternatives and drawing on previous experiences should identify the sub-goals. If alternatives cannot be found from personal experience, the person could seek alternative perspectives from family and friends or professionals. Problem solving involves goal planning and action.

Emotion-focused coping

This approach is more about dealing with the feeling of stress. It is suggested that this may be the best way of managing stress when there is no way of finding a solution to the problem. This could involve trying to see a positive side, keeping busy, and focusing on other things using meditation and exercise. Sometimes people use both coping strategies at the same time. They are working through sub-goals at the same time as managing their emotions.

Mike would appear to be using an emotion-focused coping strategy by trying to make himself feel better by taking a step back from the situation. Unfortunately, Mike's response is not improving his situation and is leading him to have ongoing problems, and he is likely to have poor health outcomes.

It may be that for Mike, given his ability to learn and his history of panic attacks, a cognitive behavioural therapeutic approach would be more helpful rather than just giving him the opportunity to choose other coping strategies.

Cognitive behavioural approaches to therapy were considered in Chapter 6.

Chapter summary

This chapter has focused on how people cope with suffering initially, by exploring what constitutes suffering and how this is relevant to nursing. This led on to considering health psychology and its usefulness to nurses when caring for those suffering. An

Continued

historical approach was taken, leading to a brief overview of mind–body medicine linked to psychoneuroimmunology. This should have offered an understanding of why mind–body medicine and a holistic approach to care was important. Health models developed by psychologists were considered, and how these might assist nurses when trying to influence behaviour change to attempt to reduce suffering and increase quality of life. Personality was also considered in relation to expectations of well-being, which recognised that although the research was limited it demonstrated that it is perhaps unhelpful to experience high expressed emotion or to attempt to totally inhibit emotional experience. The chapter concluded with a case study of nursing care of a person suffering from pain, including an explanation of the underlying theory, and a case study of a person suffering from extreme stress. The coping strategies identified in the pain case study and the stress case study could all be accessed and used by nurses, as well as being applicable to the people for whom nurses care.

References

Ajzen I. (1988) *Attitudes, Personality and Behaviour*. Milton Keynes: Open University Press.

Carlson N.R. (1998) *Physiology of Behaviour*, 9th edition. Needham Heights, MA: Allyn and Bacon.

Evans P., Hucklebridge F. & Clow A. (2000) *Mind, Immunity and Health, The Science of Psychoneuroimmunology*. London: Free Associates Books.

Ferrell B.R. (1996) *Suffering*, p. 5. Sudbury, MA: Jones and Bartlett Publishers.

Folkman S. & Lazarus R.S. (1991) The concept of coping. In Monat A. & Lazarus R.S. (eds) *Stress and Coping: An Anthology*, 3rd edition. New York: Columbia University Press.

Gross R. (2001) *Psychology: The Science of Mind and Behaviour*, 4th edition. London: Hodder & Stoughton.

Lazarus R.S. (1966) *Psychological Stress and the Coping Process*. New York: McGraw-Hill.

Melzack R. & Wall P.D. (1982) *The Challenge of Pain*. New York: Basic Books.

Morrison V. & Bennett P. (2006) *An Introduction to Health Psychology*. London: Pearson Prentice Hall.

Naidoo J. & Wills J. (2001) *Health Studies, An Introduction*. Basingstoke: Palgrave.

Ogden J. (2000) *Health Psychology: A textbook*, 2nd edition, p. 292. Milton Keynes: Open University.

Prochaska J.O. & Diclemente C.C. (1984) *The Transtheoretical Approach: Crossing Traditional Boundaries of Change*. Homeward, IL: Irwin.

Roberts R., Towell T. & Golding J.F. (2001) *Foundations of Health Psychology*. Basingstoke: Palgrave.

Schwarzer R. (1992) Self efficacy in the adoption and maintenance of health behaviours: theoretical approaches and a new model. In Schwarzer R. (ed.) *Self Efficacy: Thought Control of Action*. Washington: Hemisphere.

Selye H. (1956) *The Stress of Life*. New York: McGraw-Hill.

Taylor S.E. (1995) *Health Psychology*, 3rd edition, p. 381. London: McGraw-Hill International Editions.

Watkins A. (1997) *Mind-Body Medicine, A Clinician's Guide to Psychoneuroimmunology*. London: Churchill Livingstone.

Index

Page numbers in *italics* refer to figures; those in **bold** to tables.